you are what you eat™

Michelle's Diary

All recipes serve one person unless otherwise stated.

you are what you eat ™

Michelle's Diary

Michelle McManus

A Celador Production as seen on Channel Four

www.youarewhatyoueat.tv

Michael O'Mara Books Limited

First published in Great Britain in 2005 by
Michael O'Mara Books Limited
9 Lion Yard
Tremadoc Road
London SW4 7NQ

A CIP catalogue record for this book is available from the British Library

ISBN (10-digit): 1-84317-192-9
ISBN (13-digit): 978-1-84317-192-8

1 3 5 7 9 10 8 6 4 2

www.mombooks.com

Designed and typeset by E-Type
Plates section design by Button Group plc

Printed and bound in Great Britain by Clays Ltd, St Ives plc

CONTENTS

ACKNOWLEDGEMENTS

I would like to thank everyone who has helped me with this book, especially:

Simon, Nicki, Charlotte Martin and everyone at 19 Management for starting me on this journey

Gillian McKeith for putting me on the right road

Claire Masters, Damon, Yvette, Amanda, Rosanna and everyone at Celador

Rick, Jeff, Joan, Deke, Alan and Alison at Sanctuary Entertainment – onwards and upwards!

My lawyer, Ann Harrison and John McGuire, lawyer at Sanctuary, for their efforts on the book deal

Emma Dickens for all those hours of torture having to listen to me

Leah and Lisa at LDA Communications

Dax Moy for inspiring me and introducing exercise and fitness to my life (even though I do call you 'the Devil'!)

Alice Theobald at Joy Goodman and Lindsey Baker for the make-up and styling

Armand Attard for the great photos

All my friends and family who have supported me my whole life

And finally, Lindsay, Chris, Kate, Alison, Hannah, Mike and everyone at Michael O'Mara Books for giving me the opportunity to tell my story and pass on what I've learned to other people in my position.

The publishers would also like to thank Alex Gazzola for his work as the nutritional consultant on this project.

PICTURE CREDITS

Pages 1–3: Michelle McManus; page 4: FremantleMedia (*above*), Michelle McManus (*below*); page 5: FremantleMedia (*above*), Theodore Wood, Camera Press London (*below*); page 6: FremantleMedia (*above*), Michelle McManus (*below*); page 7: www.expresspictures.com (*above*), Rex Features (*below*); page 8: FremantleMedia; page 9: David Rankin, Camera Press London (*above*), Rex Features (*below*); page 10: BIG Pictures; pages 11–13: courtesy of Celador Productions; page 14: courtesy of Celador Productions (*above*), Mark Anderson / Rex Features (*below*); pages 15–16: www.armandattard.com.

CLOTHES CREDITS

Front cover, right: wrap jumper and jeans: Anna Scholz

Back cover: sequin bolero – Wallis; camisole top – Dorothy Perkins

Plate section page 15, top: black dress – New Look; knitted shrug with satin trim – Linea at House of Fraser

Plate section page 15, bottom, and page 16: chiffon beaded top – Evans; black trousers – Wallis

INTRODUCTION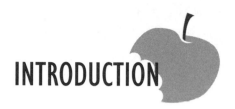

It's Saturday, 20 December 2003. The final of *Pop Idol*. Pretty much all of 2003 has been taken up with the show and now it's the climax of the whole competition. I'd thought maybe I'd be this year's token fat girl, but here I am, sitting in a dressing room in Fountain Studios, Wembley, at a quarter to ten in the morning while Mark Rhodes, the other finalist, is downstairs doing his soundcheck.

I'm watching Mark on the monitor and I'm thinking, 'I'm in the final of the biggest talent show in the UK and I've got a 50 per cent chance of winning!' It's a freezing cold morning and I'm feeling self-conscious because my hair had been dyed back to black to give me a different look for that week.

There's a tap on the door and someone says, 'Right, Michelle. Come on down and do your soundcheck.' And all I can think is, 'This is the last time I'm going to be here. This is the last time I'm going to have a soundcheck.' Suddenly I'm not thinking about winning any more, I'm thinking, 'This ride's coming to an end. No more Saturdays. No more living in the big house. What's going to happen now? My life's going to change after this.' Even *Pop Idol* itself is a security blanket – we've been doing it for twelve weeks. It's become a routine.

The soundcheck goes well. Afterwards, I go back upstairs, and Mark and I mess around for a bit.

Everyone is so, so excited. I'm sure they're all laying bets on who's going to win, but they have to be really diplomatic about it because they can't show any favouritism.

Next we get our hair and make-up done and before I know it, it's 6.30 at night and the show is starting. I'm not allowing myself to think I'll win the final, because it's so up in the air: there were straw polls on *GMTV* and *This Morning* – the first said I was going to win, and the second that Mark would.

The desire to win is coming over me strongly now, but although I've been shaking all day, the nerves are starting to get out of control. I've hardly eaten a thing today.

And now Mark and I are standing by the stage and the *Pop Idol* music comes on, and Mark is saying, 'Good luck, babe,' and I'm saying, 'Yeah, good luck to you, too.'

I can see the audience is packed and I can see the four judges sitting there – Simon Cowell, Pete Waterman, Dr Fox and Nicki Chapman – and twenty-five of my family and friends. My dad is dressed up as Rod Stewart, with leopard-print tights. He's dressed up every week I've been on. Whatever the show's theme – whether it was the Beatles or Elton John songs we had to sing, for example – he and my uncles always came along looking like that artist.

So, cue music; cue the show's hosts – Ant and Dec – running on and doing their introductions. Then we walk on, waving to the millions of viewers out there.

First off, Mark stays onstage and sings 'All This Time'. We both have to sing the same song in this first round, then we get to choose our next two numbers ourselves.

Standing by the stage, watching Mark, I'm starting to think tactically, song by song. He's doing a great job, but I like my version of this tune better.

It's my turn next. I give it everything I've got, then come off and change while Mark sings 'She's Like The Wind' – his money song. I'm thinking, 'Bastard', as all the women in the country melt.

During the previous week, Simon Cowell had advised me to change my next song from 'Don't Be A Stranger' to 'On The Radio'. I'd said, 'But ballads are my thing,' and he came right back with, 'I'm telling you. Get some pyrotechnics in there and show them you can be a pop star.'

So I blast out 'On The Radio' – with my pyrotechnics!

Next comes the comments from the judges: 'You could really do this tonight,' and 'This could really be your night' – both from Simon.

And 'Oh, I think Mark's giving you a run for your money,' from Pete Waterman.

Pete never liked me.

I go over and sit with Ant and Dec for my post-song interview. 'What do you think?' they ask me.

'Even now, all the press are saying I can't win it and I shouldn't win it. But why not? Why shouldn't I win it?' I reply. I start crying, though I'm trying to hold it back, and all the while I'm thinking, 'Just let the public decide. If I'm not supposed to win I won't win.'

Then I come back on and sing 'The Meaning Of Love'. It goes brilliantly.

Mark and I spend the next hour off-air, cacking ourselves. We sit and shake, and the two of us can't even talk to each other. It's a nightmare. I just want everything to be over.

By the time we go back down for the announcement there are 17 million viewers waiting to see the result. I'm just staring at Ant and Dec, wanting them to give me a sign that it's me. If you look at my face in the recording of the show, you'll see that I'm deathly white at this point.

'And the winner of *Pop Idol* 2003 is . . .'

I look out and see my dad in his Rod Stewart wig; all my friends and family are crying by now, waiting to hear the outcome. They've got up every Saturday morning at five o'clock, caught the 5.50 a.m. train from Glasgow to London, and twenty-five of them have been on this train for twelve weeks solid. Virgin has ended up giving them all free tickets.

'. . . Michelle!'

And total silence. I can't hear anything – no cheers, no applause, just that name ringing through my head, and my own thoughts: 'Michelle, you've won.' The next minute I'm nearly down on my knees because my balance has gone.

Mark grabs me and holds me up, saying, 'Miche, you've done it! You've done it!'

My family are all jumping up and down and crying. And I'm thinking, 'I haven't just done this for myself. I've done this for them too.'

Then I have to go and sing again, and – to my complete surprise – all the final twelve *Pop Idol* contestants join me on-stage too.

I look down and Pete Waterman is storming off set because I've won. I've got 6.5 million votes and Mark's got 4.5 million.

And I'm standing with all this confetti around me, thinking, 'How did an overweight, working-class girl from Glasgow get here?' It's like a movie. It's like falling.

My life changed completely from that point. From then on it was promotion, promotion, promotion, publicity, singles, albums coming out, and life became like a rollercoaster ride.

You allow yourself to be duped into thinking that that's

it – you're made now and nothing bad's ever going to happen to you again. You go from zero to hero in about six months and you're up in the clouds. You don't get much higher than 17 million viewers – and the only way is down. That's the celeb's life.

The rest of the night I won was spent with my family; I couldn't even drink because I was so hyper. Afterwards we were taken back to the house in Regent's Park, north London, where I'd been living for the previous twelve weeks with the other finalists. Mark was amazing about it, such a gentleman. He just kept hugging me and telling me how well I'd done. I don't know whether I'd have been that gracious if he'd won.

I lay awake the whole night. When I was on my own, at 2 a.m., I even cried because I was so happy – though I'm not an idiot and I knew things wouldn't be this way for ever. I had no idea what lay ahead of me, and that sense of the unknown was what scared me the most.

When I went home to Glasgow I was told I couldn't go back to my mum and dad's house because it had turned into a media circus there. So I booked my entire family into a hotel – they had to be smuggled out in vans in the middle of the night and taken to the hotel, where we spent our Christmas. Journalists even went to my gran's house on Christmas Day with a Christmas cake. Didn't they have better things to do?

Only one thing clouded that winning night for me: the 'dress' I wore made me acutely aware of my weight. It was basically a black bag with green netting around it. I had told the stylist that I just wanted a nice black evening dress. 'You can't go wrong,' I thought to myself. 'Do you need my measurements?' I asked him.

'No, no, no, no, no,' he replied. 'I've been styling you for twelve weeks!'

On the day of the live final the stylist was late in arriving and I started to get really nervous. We were due to do a full dress rehearsal at 5 p.m., but by 4.30 p.m. there was still no sign of the dress. In the end, the stylist showed up at 4.45 p.m. I took one look at the outfit he'd chosen for me and broke down in tears. I'll never forget it: it was this black tent – and strapless.

'Are you trying to make me look ten times bigger than I am?' I sobbed. 'I'm not going on national TV with nothing round my arms!'

So he cut some of the netting off the underskirt and put it round my shoulders. It was blue. How I won that show wearing that dress, I'll never know – I should have been shot.

Afterwards, Simon told me, 'You were fab – but burn the dress!'

Apart from that, I was as happy as a person could be. I remember thinking that I could now pay off my parents' mortgage. Nothing was further from my mind than losing weight at that stage. Every couple of months the thought of shedding a few pounds would cross my mind, but then so would changing my hair colour – or my boyfriend.

In any case, I was too busy to stop and think about anything as mundane as going on a diet, not when there were so many exciting things going on all around me. It was certainly a surreal time: I got a letter from Gordon Brown after I won – handwritten. It said, 'We're so proud of you and what you've done for Scotland. We think you're amazing and we'll buy the album.' Mo Mowlam mentioned me in a piece for the *Independent* too.

It was my granny who started me singing – the same granny who put my weight down to a thyroid problem, bless her. I went to playgroup when I was three years old and I was a terrible show-off – I have four younger sisters (and they all sing too), but I was the worst, the family party-piece. My mother tells this story about how she was called in by the teacher one day to discuss me. A large group of children had been trying to read a story, apparently, and I had marched up to the front of the class and started singing 'Down In The Jungle Where Nobody Goes'. I also sang 'Nobody Likes Me, Everybody Hates Me, I Think I'll Go and Eat Worms'. They were both songs my granny had taught me.

The teacher tried in vain to get me to shut up and sit down. It didn't work, though – I even started doing a bit of a dance for them.

'You have to control your child,' the teacher told Mum later.

'She sings everywhere. I don't know what to do with her,' Mum replied.

Before *Pop Idol* I had a full-time job in Glasgow as an events manager for the Marriott chain of hotels, but I always thought of myself as a singer – though not necessarily a professional. I was confident that I could sing, and I always had it in my head that one day something would happen and I would make it. Everyone aspires to be someone and I always had the attitude that something would come along. So, as much as winning *Pop Idol* was a shock, I had almost semi-prepared myself. I had been practising my autograph since I was five years old! Maybe I voodooed everyone.

My schooldays were the best of my life. Honest they were. One guy who was my flatmate after I left school made twenty grand out of claiming to the tabloids that I was bullied at school because of my size. He said I didn't have any boyfriends as a result of my weight. I never believed that anyone would do such a thing until I experienced it for myself after *Pop Idol*. If you've ever wondered who would be mostly likely to kiss 'n' tell if you got famous, it's that guy you've forgotten all about who just crossed your path for a couple of years.

It's a bit of a sad story really, because I was nineteen and I'd fallen for this guy, big style. It was never reciprocated. We kissed a few times, but nothing major. Nevertheless, it still hurt when I read the lies he told about me. It wasn't just him, either. There was another guy who jumped on the Michelle-was-bullied-at-school-and-she-nearly-had-a-nervous-breakdown bandwagon too and who sold his story to a tabloid. Neither of them even went to my school!

In fact, I wasn't that big at primary school, although I've always been bigger than my four sisters. It was in my teens that I really started piling the weight on, and if it was for emotional reasons, I wasn't aware of them at the time. Gillian McKeith – the woman who finally turned round my approach to eating – always tries to deal first with what she calls 'the emotional crap' when she meets someone she's going to help. But as far as I know there really weren't any issues with me – I was just addicted to junk food and alcohol. Simple as that. I've really searched my soul and I can't come up with any other reason.

All I can think is that I have a bit of an addictive personality, which is both my best asset and my worst enemy. Not so good when I was turning down Mum's home cooking in favour of McDonald's, or going out binge drinking, but handy when it comes to being focused on my career – or committing to the *You Are What You Eat* healthy-eating plan.

Perhaps the problem was that my family never put me under any pressure about my weight. No one ever even mentioned it. I knew from looking at them that I was different from my sisters, but my parents were just so amazing, always saying, 'You look beautiful.' Maybe my mother secretly worried about my weight, but she never said so. I think she just saw that I was genuinely happy. And how many teenagers are genuinely happy with themselves?

People don't believe me when I say that I don't have any memories of questioning my weight or being upset about it. I do remember one occasion, when I was eleven or twelve years old and I'd just got really big, and I went on a school trip to York. It was summer, so I had shorts on, and I remember my thighs rubbing together and going all red. I was in agony and didn't know who to turn to or what to do. So I phoned my mum. 'Why don't you buy a wee tub of Vaseline and that will help you. It happens to lots of people, don't worry,' she told me. I was really embarrassed and couldn't wear shorts for the rest of the week because I had these red blotches on my legs, but perhaps what I should have been embarrassed about was the fact that my legs were so much bigger than the other girls'.

I'm no expert, but as I understand it anorexia is being down on yourself, seeing yourself as big even though you're not, and telling yourself you need to lose weight even when you don't. I was the opposite. No one was telling me there was a problem and I was so up on myself that I couldn't see it. It would have only been human for my parents to worry, but it wasn't as if I was moping about the house or anything, so they left me to it. So many kids have got a complex about themselves and my parents believed – rightly, I think – that the most important thing is to make sure you are happy in your own skin.

If I ever have a big kid, I think I'll want to instil a similar sense of self-worth in my child as my mum did with me, although I'd like to think that things might be different knowing what I know now about healthy eating. You've got to remember that it's only in the past five years that people have really got to grips with re-educating themselves about food. Twenty years ago, when I was a child, it was all about plain, home-cooked meals: mince and potatoes. Nothing fancy – the important thing was that it was cheap and filling and tasted good. Mine was a big, working-class family on a budget – knowing about omega-3 fatty acids and 'good' and 'bad' fats didn't come into it.

I'd like to think that when I'm a mum I'll bring good, healthy, nutritious food to the table – and teach my kids about food in the way that I've been educated by *You Are What You Eat* – but I won't deny them anything. I think kids need treats and sweets, but just not on tap. And no junk food.

Don't get me wrong, though. Mum was no pushover. She'd put some home-cooked food on the table and I'd say, 'I don't want that, I want a chippy.' And she'd come right back at me with, 'Absolutely not, Michelle McManus! You'll eat what's put in front of you!'

Dad would say, 'There's children starving in Africa.'

'They don't have a chippy,' I'd reply. Then I'd just pick at the food and sneak out to the chippy later.

There are no excuses as to why I became so overweight. It wasn't that we didn't get enough attention. Although there were five of us, we all got loads of attention. I was the oldest, but I don't remember being the only child and then feeling jealous when my first sibling (Lynsey) came along, because I was only a year and a half older than her – as far as I was concerned, she was always there. Lynsey is twenty-three and works for British Telecom as a manager; Laura's twenty and she's a hairdresser working for one of the top salons in Glasgow; Maria's seventeen and sitting her A levels. She wants to be a psychologist. Kerry (thirteen going on thirty) has recently informed the family that not only is she going to get tattoos, but she also reckons she's getting her tongue pierced. Which is why she's been grounded until she turns eighteen. She says the entire family's 'gay'.

I do crave attention, but I always got it at home. If anything, I wanted a bit of peace and quiet in my house. That was why I moved out when I was nineteen. I couldn't breathe.

Jenni Murray, from Radio 4's *Woman's Hour*, said that I have the 'Wit of the Big Woman', the one who gets the joke in before anyone else does. She might be right, I don't know. But I don't make jokes about my weight that much. I think you inherit your humour from your family. My dad's very funny and we were brought up on *Blackadder*, *Fawlty Towers*, *Only Fools and Horses* and *Not the Nine O'Clock News* because that was the kind of stuff Dad loved. Oh well, better to be called witty than big and bubbly, I suppose.

One thing that is definitely a myth perpetuated by the press is that I'm a diva who demands chocolate before going on MTV. The fact is I've never been into chocolate or sweets – it was always the savoury stuff: pizza, chips, burgers. And no, I don't demand pizzas before going onstage either.

My sisters and friends ate junk food as well, but the difference between them and me is that I didn't automatically burn it off. I can go away for a weekend with the girls and put on half a stone. The upside, I've since found, is that with a bit of effort I can lose it easily too. You know, I have nothing but sympathy for people who are trying to lose weight. I love food. I really enjoy eating food. You don't want to give up what you like. And you don't need to be severely emotionally scarred to find food comforting.

A year before going on *Pop Idol*, I won six talent shows. It was good money – I won six grand – but I spent it all on going out and boozing. I didn't use any of the money for anything useful. I used to do the talent shows at night in working-men's clubs – it was just like *Phoenix Nights*, but I loved it. The characters you'd find in those places were unbelievable. There was this one woman who was the epitome of a club singer – beautiful looking, about sixty. I've never heard anything like her version of 'The Power Of Love': '. . . Caws ayam yer leardeee . . . ,' she would sing in the broadest Scots accent going.

I love clubland, all the bitching and the backstabbing. And all the competitions are rigged, I'm sure they are. I always felt that there were people in Glasgow who wouldn't let me win their club's talent show because I didn't look the part in the photographs. Either that or I was just crap and didn't realize it.

I'd get so far, perhaps into the semi-final, and then all of a sudden get knocked out for no reason. I remember singing in one club when this guy had forgotten his words and was singing off-key, and yet he still went through to the next round. I remember thinking, 'Something's not right here.'

Ah yes – seriously dodgy decisions, sparkly jackets and

wigs – it was a great time. I started when I was sixteen, nearly ten years ago, and in those days there just weren't the fashionable clothes for the larger woman that there are today. I used to look simply horrendous – thick, unplucked eyebrows, bad make-up and perm, a middle-aged navy dress with a pink cardigan. 'Or perhaps a purple, stretchy, Lycra dress cut at the diagonal from the knee to the floor, madam?' Don't forget to accessorize with big block heels and team it with an old man's black cardigan.

I still keep in touch with some of the keyboard guys on the circuit and they make me laugh. They say, 'Nothing's changed up here. We've still got Bessie singing "The Power Of Love".' But I'd do it again in a second for charity or to help mates out.

I didn't even know the auditions were happening for the first *Pop Idol* in 2002 – which obviously drove me mental when I found out. I didn't watch it at first because I was so angry I'd missed out and so jealous of the people that were on there. It was unbelievable to me: here was this TV show willing to open its doors to anyone – not just skinny people, not just beautiful people, not even just great singers. You could be anyone from anywhere and after the public had got to know you and your voice it would be up to them to decide whether they wanted you to be a singer or not.

When it came to the final, everyone thought Gareth Gates was going to win. But – as we all know now – Will Young surprised everyone by triumphing on the night. Now OK, Will's not overweight, but he's not everyone's idea of a pop star either, and that was quite inspirational for me. I thought, 'Wait a minute. This guy's different. He's not a normal Pop

Idol and yet he's won this show.' It made me really want to have a go the following year. I thought I was capable of being a good contender, and perhaps even reaching the final stage, or at the very least getting some feedback and useful pointers that would help me with my club singing. But because of my weight I thought there was absolutely no chance I was ever going to win.

The night Will won, when a phone number came up on screen, I applied – and didn't hear a thing for a year and a half. Then I got a letter asking me to come along for an audition. Of course, I went along wearing black, because I wanted to look as thin as I possibly could. People wearing black always think they look three stone lighter.

I remember that audition really clearly. There they were, the three judges – Simon Cowell, Nicki Chapman and Pete Waterman – and I could sense straight away that they were all thinking, 'What is this girl thinking of?' Perhaps I was just being ultra-paranoid. Then I sang, 'Because You Love Me'. Simon had said beforehand that the song was one of his favourites. Afterwards, though, Nicki was the first to speak.

'Look, you don't look like a Pop Idol, but I think you've got a great voice and I'd love to see you through,' she told me. She was to be a key part of my career from that moment on.

Pete Waterman went on this five-minute rant. 'You're not a Pop Idol. You will never be a Pop Idol. It doesn't mean you're not a good singer, but you will never win this show. You're not a Pop Idol.' They played that footage when I won the competition, which was funny.

So it was all down to Simon Cowell.

'I'm going to put you through. I like you,' he said.

As I ran out to Granny, who was waiting outside, to tell her I'd made it to the next round, I remember feeling beside myself with excitement, but so sick at the same time, thinking, 'What have I let myself in for here?' I knew I was overweight and I knew that if I was in the public eye I was going to get slaughtered. I had lived with myself for a long time and was completely comfortable in my own skin, but I also knew how society looks upon overweight people.

Then I got to the final-fifty stage. I was performing in the first group of ten. The week before the live shows they had shown me reaching the final hundred and I'd said 'Thank you' when I was told I'd got through. But they edited it so that Simon Cowell was nodding his head as though I was saying thank you to him. So the papers were full of how Simon had let his guard down for once – when actually the person I had been thanking was Nicki!

I won that first live show with over 30 per cent of the votes, which was the biggest majority of the whole series. I was growing more and more scared, though. Was this really what I wanted to do with my life? I'd always thought that the final-fifty stage would be as far as I was going to get.

Then we were the final twelve, with the addition of two more performers from the 'wild card' round. I thought the others were all really talented, but the person I got on best with was Brian Ormond, the blond Irish guy, because he always looked at me as a serious contender, and not just a token fat girl. I'm not saying they all did that, but generally the group either thought I had no chance or that I'd win out of sympathy. By the time we'd got to the final stage, everyone wanted it really badly.

Susanne Manning (the beautiful, curvy blonde whom Simon Cowell said he wanted to marry) and I had a turbulent relationship because it was alleged in the press that she'd said, 'I'm not standing by that fat cow.' Whether or not she did I've no idea, but either way we clashed. I don't even know if the clash was real now because it was such a pressurized situation back then. We get on fine these days.

There was a lovely, smiley, blonde girl called Kim Gee, my partner in crime, who got knocked out really early on, and that put to rest my fear that they were just keeping us on because we were both big. Although Kim was a fabulous singer, I thought, 'Maybe it's not just a sympathy vote; maybe people are voting for me because I can sing.' It helped me to start believing in myself more and more.

As for Mark Rhodes, our relationship was not all professionalism to the end. It was me who started calling him Cheesy Mark. In the final week, everywhere he went I sent him cheese. And as I was always interviewed first, each time I would leave the interviewer with a block of cheese to give him. At the end he recycled all the cheese, put it in a paint-ball gun and paint-balled my tour bus with it!

By the time we got down to the last three – it was between myself, Sam Nixon and Mark Rhodes – we still got on like a house on fire. I love those two boys because it was just such an intense time and we'd come so far together; no one else can ever understand what we went through.

Once all the other finalists had been knocked out they were able to detach themselves from the programme. They were all great about me winning. Although I expected to get voted off every week, I don't know how I'd have reacted towards the others if I *had* been voted off.

I keep in touch with almost all the final twelve, especially since we went on tour together after the series finished. I have to say, I did struggle with the touring. Ten dates with three weeks' rehearsal – it was exhausting. I wasn't fit enough for it. I ate junk food continuously, even though there was catering provided. Afterwards I felt I should have done something to prepare myself. I was at my biggest and I looked humungous onstage. Trying to dance and sing at the same time left me constantly out of breath.

POP IDOL CLASS OF 2003 – WHERE ARE THEY NOW?

- Marc Dillon has had a baby and is doing gigs up and down the country.
- Brian Ormond is hugely successful and works for RTE as a TV presenter.
- Susanne Manning is getting married and works for BBC radio.
- Chris Hide was doing Butlins with Bucks Fizz and is trying to get a record deal.
- Kim Gee is one of my best friends from the show and has had a couple of good auditions in the West End. She's doing some dance tracks and backing vocals.
- I think Roxanne Cooper is working on an R&B album.
- Andy Scott Lee has just finished doing *Totally Scott Lee* on MTV and has a single coming out next year.
- Mark Rhodes and Sam Nixon present *Top of the Pops Reloaded*.

Bizarrely, I got more presents and fan mail than any of the other girls: diamond earrings, a diamond bracelet, flowers. It was hysterical. There were all these stunning-looking girls and I was the only one who received any serious fan mail. At one point, a security guard at Dixons even got down on one knee and asked me to marry him.

Although I'm used to performing onstage, singing to millions of people on *Pop Idol* is obviously a different thing altogether. I was a nervous wreck every time I went out there. One time I was in such a state that I puked on one of the backstage crew – classy. Bless him, he just stood there and said, 'It's OK.'

Vocal coaching – every Thursday and on the day of the show – reassured some of us. We'd do warm-ups, but I found the whole thing extremely embarrassing: everyone going 'Meee-meee-meee-meee-meee' and making all these strange sounds. And I couldn't even tell the difference in my voice after I tried it. But John and Cece, the vocal coaches, say if you don't sing for a while your vocal chords close up.

Nowadays I'm appalling with my voice. I don't do any vocal training or exercises, and I really should. When I record, I just go in and sing the song a couple of times and whatever comes out, comes out. If I know I've got a big gig the next day I don't go out the night before, but that's about it. There's a sound-check before and that does for me. Other than that I have a ginger and lemon tea or something. You're not supposed to take a freezing cold drink before singing. Before I started the *You Are What You Eat* plan I would have had a brandy as well, but not any more, obviously.

Loads of people do take care of their voices with throat medicines and sprays. Some people even put these face inhaler things on, which clear their nose, ears and throat – but they're not for me. I believe people like Mariah Carey don't talk for a couple of hours before they sing. I can't imagine not speaking for that long.

Since I've lost weight, my voice has changed. I think people will be quite surprised to hear the new album, because it sounds different. I don't know whether it's better or worse, but I think on the whole the bigger you are, the better your voice is – look at opera singers. I don't know why. Maybe it's because you have pressure on your lungs, which gives a different sound, or something. I think I've lost that deep, soul thing I had. Although having said that, your voice usually deepens as you get older anyway. I sound different now from how I did as a teenager. I heard Kate Bush's comeback single recently; I'm a huge Kate Bush fan, and you can really tell the difference in her voice between her new material and the songs she was singing twenty years ago.

In August 2005, Simon Cowell was reported in the press as saying that I was over and that he only supported me back in 2003 because there was no one else – which couldn't have been much further from 'she's funny and optimistic and a kick up the backside for the music industry,' which was what he said during *Pop Idol*. But I've got to admit that he was the major reason I won the show, because he backed me so strongly. In fact, I didn't realize how much he'd supported me until I watched the programmes again.

That said, he only gave his support up to a point. On the night I won *Pop Idol* he took me and my mum to one side and said, 'Don't worry, we're going to take care of you' – and we never saw him again after that evening! Perhaps he meant the people who worked on the show as a whole would take care of me. It's true, I did make some lifelong friends there.

I remember some MSPs, including Tommy Sheridan,

accusing Simon of wrecking kids' confidence on the show, but Simon is what he is. He's an A&R man who's created this whole persona for himself for *Pop Idol* and *The X Factor*. He is the guy who has taken America by storm with his sharp and slightly insulting comments, and, let's not forget, his wicked charm! When you're up in front of Simon Cowell, you know he's not just going to say something nice for the sake of it.

Those MSPs also said that people should be judged on their singing talent and not on preconceived images. God love them for trying, but Pete Waterman – whose comments prompted the MSP's remarks – is old school and entitled to say what he thinks. And he's right – my second single hardly sold.

The only way people – including Simon – could relate to my size was by comparing me to Alison Moyet or Mama Cass. Both are compliments, because both those singers have fantastic voices, but let's face it, they were mentioned because they were the only overweight pop stars people could think of. That's not to say that appearance is always everything. Dido's attractive but her music is the first thing you think of, before her looks.

Somehow this topic got me into trouble on one occasion. The *Mirror* ran a piece stating that I'd said something to the effect of 'You don't have to be good-looking to be successful – look at Meat Loaf.' He held up the spread at a gig saying, 'Who does this f**king bitch think she is?' Actually, I'd said, 'You don't have to conform to be a success – look at Meat Loaf, he's a sex symbol.' Eventually he got the gist of what I'd really said and sent me a massive bouquet of flowers to apologize – perhaps with some encouragement from his management.

Simon said that, as with Darius, the whole of Scotland was behind me, but talk of 'the Scotland Vote' makes me laugh. I'm very patriotic but there are 6 million people in Scotland and

7½ million people in London alone – so I'm not sure how this tiny wee country can be expected to make such a difference.

Perhaps the biggest lesson I learned from that time was about how the British tabloid press works. I know there's a lot of talk about this from people in the public eye, and a lot of bitching about it from those who are happy to court it when the publicity is good – but you have to experience it to believe it. And I'm such an easy target – after all, it doesn't take much to call someone fat. I can't expect to be in the public eye and for the media not to comment on my size.

The people I most admire are those who get knocked down and get back up again. Like Jade Goody from *Big Brother*, or Darius, who couldn't have been knocked more by the press, but who held his head high and came back and turned it all around for himself. That demands respect. The last I read he was on a catwalk at a New York fashion show – you can't argue with that.

What the tabloids said about Jade Goody was disgusting. *Big Brother* contestants are driven mental because it's such a confined space, and while they're in the house the programme-makers fill them up with drink. How they don't lose their minds in there I have no idea. I'm a huge Jade Goody fan. Everyone knows who she is and she's worth a fortune now.

I don't have a problem with people being famous for being famous. After all, somebody's obviously buying the magazines that feature these celebrities; somebody's obviously interested. They're providing some sort of service. I really like Jordan, for example. Bloody clever woman – a self-made millionaire. OK, some people may think she's tacky, but she's a product of what we want as a society. People want to see this woman with huge boobs, decked out in miniskirts. A ridiculous number of people bought

OK! magazine to see her wedding photographs. Good on her. Go lady.

You have to remember with journalism that it's only one person's opinion – it's just that they have the privilege of communicating that opinion to millions of people. Dominic Mohan didn't hold back in his opinions of me in the *Sun*. He said, 'Don't get me wrong, Michelle can sing, but I'm sorry though, she ain't no Pop Idol . . . You just wouldn't, would you?' He went on to say that people become Pop Idols because you either want to be them or dream of sleeping with them. I know what he's getting at, but he was wrong in my case. Or perhaps more men want to bed larger ladies than are letting on . . .

In fact, the majority of my fan base is made up of gay men or young girls. And women like me because I'm not the kind of woman who would steal your man. Also, I think women like women who can speak their mind, who've got something about them.

I wonder if Dominic is right to speak for others when he tells them who he fancies. I fancy all sorts of people – I don't give a stuff whether they're big, small, whatever. Judging from my own experience, men do fancy big women, it's just that it's not cool to be seen to do so. You're not supposed to fancy the fat girl in the corner, it doesn't look good in front of your mates. But it doesn't stop men secretly finding us big girls attractive. Certainly, I've never had any problems pulling men. Most of the guys I've been out with were gorgeous-looking, and I was a size 26 for the majority of that time. They didn't like me because I looked great in a bikini, but because I could hold my own and have a laugh, and if people wanted to have a conversation with me I could answer them in a reasonably intelligent manner. It's true what they say. Being comfortable with yourself is very attractive.

Sharon Hendry, editor of the *Sun*'s women's section, certainly got my vote when she said, 'We're bored, bored, bored of bare-skinned bonebags banging out bad vocals.' I think she was pointing out that it was nice to see someone 'normal' on TV. Let's face it, many of the women in Hollywood and the pop industry are abnormally thin on the whole. I don't have an issue with that, but it doesn't do much for an ordinary woman's self-esteem to look at a magazine or a TV screen and try to work out why these celebs are so thin and successful, and they're not. It dominates every magazine. I can sit in a pub on a Friday night and guarantee that there are tables full of women talking about their weight. It's not their fault, it's just that that's what everyone talks about. Personally, I don't care who's skinny and who's fat. This is obviously why I let myself get so big, but it honestly doesn't concern me. I don't care whether people are a size 6 or a 16, though of course when your weight starts to affect your health – if you're constantly out of breath, or you've got knee problems, or more serious obesity-related conditions like heart disease or stroke – then that's a different matter.

And women have become their own worst enemies. How many times has a woman looked you up and down when you go into a bar? Some female journalists are no different. One, who is overweight herself, got really vindictive about me, talking about me eating cream cakes all the time. This woman is reasonably intelligent, so it must be her choice to be overweight herself, yet she has a go at me about my lack of self-control. I admire strong women who have something to say for themselves, but in this case it's not just double standards, it's lazy journalism. She also said that overweight women are constantly ignored, but I've never been ignored. That might be her personal experience, but it's not mine.

The other thing that makes me laugh is these journalists who criticize people for having surgery or using airbrushed photos of themselves, when their own picture byline is about twenty years old. Well, put an up-to-date picture of yourself up there, then!

The *Daily Star* claimed I'd said that fame scares me, but I never thought about fame. I never craved it. What scared me was the fact that the media builds you up to a point where you can't get any higher: you're on the front cover of all the magazines; you're water-cooler chat at work. Unless you're pretty stupid, before too long you start to think, 'Where do I go from here?' And, of course, where you go is down again. You learn that lesson really quickly. I knew it was coming.

It's amazing how strongly people in the media start to feel about you too, people who've never even met you and should have better things to think about. I heard that one DJ said, 'For God's sake, stop buying this record. We cannot let this fat bitch get to Number One.' The radio station was flooded with complaints, and he was taken off air and suspended. I remember thinking, 'You don't even know me. Why do you care? How can me being overweight offend you so much? You're on the radio, you don't even see the faces of the people whose music you're playing. And it should be all about the music.'

It wasn't just the tabloids that got involved, though. Lesley Garrett criticized *Pop Idol* in the *Daily Telegraph* for encouraging young people to think they can shortcut any training and go straight to fame and fortune. I love Lesley Garrett and was disappointed by this comment, because if she'd watched the show she'd have seen artists singing live consistently in front of 10 million people every Saturday night for three months. I didn't do it Lesley's way; I didn't fight tooth and nail for a record deal. But whether I fight tooth and nail before it or after it isn't really the point. I was up onstage singing live every single week for twelve solid weeks – and with all those things they said about me in the press going on in the background at the same time. I don't see that as being an easy route. Anyway, it's not the route, it's what you do when you get there that counts. And people who criticize *Pop Idol* overlook the most obvious thing of all: it's a talent show – a format as old as the hills.

So I expected criticism from the papers, but I did sometimes wish it was more about my voice and less about my weight. If people want to slag me off for not being a great singer, I can accept that. But the press obsession with me losing weight began as far back as September 2003. The auditions for *Pop Idol* had begun in May, and between then and September nothing happened with the filming. During that time I lost almost 2 stone, but it was nothing to do with wanting to be pop-star-shaped. I was attending a friend's wedding, and like every woman who's going to be a bridesmaid I wanted to lose a couple of pounds and look OK. I never vowed to go on a crash diet, which was what they said in the press at the time.

At around the same time, the *Daily Telegraph* said of pop stars that 'unfortunately, it's about having the right look – which really means the same look'. Although I had the second highest-selling single that year, I kind of agree – my career didn't really go anywhere afterwards. And because this was what the press had been waiting for, they jumped on it. Because of this backlash, my career really did die a death. Much as I hate to admit it, you can't be a pop star and be overweight. It just doesn't work. I've tried.

Then we were in talks about doing another single and I

weighed myself and thought, 'I don't give a stuff whether I never do another single again, I've just got to get myself sorted.' For the first time in my life I didn't care about music. But I don't think losing weight is a fast track to success. There are no guarantees in the music industry.

Publicity's not funny when it hurts those around you – and it'll happen eventually, if you're in the public eye. On one occasion, my mother got a phone call from a guy saying he was from my then management, 19. He told her I'd been admitted to hospital having had a drug overdose. She rang me up to discover I was in the pub with a couple of people from *Pop Idol*. The caller had been a journalist, and that weekend in the paper a story broke that I was living on my own eating TV dinners for one. At that point I had a four-bedroomed house and five of us were living together because Roxanne from the show was staying with us too. The papers said I was depressed and suicidal. In fact, I was having an absolute ball. I was out every night and having a relationship with a lovely guy.

But by far the worst time was when my elderly aunt had cancer. The family had elected not to tell her yet, but somehow a tabloid hack found out, went to her door and told her instead. They took her a bouquet of flowers saying they were from me, and she was just a little old lady, so she let them in. She died later that year and I couldn't even go to the funeral because the photographers said they'd be there and they would have ruined it.

Occasionally it's your turn to worry for the journalists, though. One Scottish sports journalist has got a column and I have no idea what that man's going to do when I reach my target size – he's going to be unemployed. He even manages to throw in a joke about me when commenting on the weekend's football scores! He's lost a couple of stone himself.

He's absolutely fascinated by me, to the point where I'm convinced he's in love with me. That's my one concern about this whole losing weight business. Will this man's family go hungry if he can't write about my weight any more? I met him once and he was terrified.

That's what I've always said about Pete Waterman: he's in love with me.

PHASE 1 — THE DIARY OF A CLUELESS DIETER

August 2004. It's nine months on from the madness of winning *Pop Idol*. The last year has been a whirlwind of meetings with record companies, promotional work, photo shoots, guest appearances and all the unreality that follows the winner of a reality-TV show. I can't say I've given my weight the slightest bit of thought. But however high you fly, eventually you have to come back down to earth. In August, I faced my own personal wake-up call.

Tuesday, 31 August 2004

22 stone

I've just had the shock of my life.

We're in the Seamill Hydro, a really posh hotel in Ayrshire, western Scotland, for Uncle Hugh's wedding. There's a set of weighing scales in the room. I was feeling really slim, dressed in black – even though it's a wedding and it's the middle of summer – and I thought I might have lost a bit of weight. So for once in my life I decided I'd weigh myself.

I'm 22 stone.

I'd always thought I was 15 or 16 stone. Having said over and over, hundreds of times, that I'm happy with myself, I can't deal with it. It's disgusting.

So I texted Nicki Chapman: 'Look, can we talk about me losing weight?'

Monday, 6 September 2004

21 stone 12 pounds

Today is the day I change my life for ever.

I love myself and everyone knows it, but at 22 stone – can't get that figure out of my head – health is a serious issue. I keep reading articles about all the diseases you're more at risk of getting if you're overweight – heart disease, type 2 diabetes, stroke, high blood pressure . . . It's time for a drastic lifestyle change. I managed to speak to Nicki on the phone this morning and she was brilliant. I've never thought about this stuff before, so I was asking her advice about how to lose weight and find a personal trainer and a dietician. I love Nicki – I can talk to her about anything.

I'm still completely hung-over from my evening out with the girls last night and paranoid from the wedding last week, and so I'm going to bed early before I drive myself crazy with thinking about this.

I'm now seeing something that Jane Moore pointed out in the *Sun* in May, when those pictures of me on the beach in Barbados came out, and which I've been denying to myself all these years: to be this big is desperately unhealthy. Still, I was gutted. I'd worked really hard and I'd gone on holiday and I didn't want to lie on the beach in jeans and a T-shirt. I wasn't hurting anybody. The pictures weren't great – they really weren't. There was one where they caught me bending over and my arse looks the size of Brazil, but I don't know what else I was supposed to do. Everyone knew what size I was – it's not as if I slipped out of my fat suit at night and I was really a size 12. For Jane Moore to say I was a beast was a bit harsh, but she's entitled to her opinion. At least I had the decency to wear a black one-piece.

Goal: to be in Barbados, in a bikini, by May 2005.

Next year I'll ring up the papers and say, 'You don't have to follow me or do anything sneaky. You can get your picture for free. I'm the one lying on the beach in a white bikini.'

Tuesday, 7 September 2004

Day 1 of the Michelle McManus 'Clueless' Diet

Breakfast: bowl of cornflakes with skimmed milk
slice of toast
Lunch: bowl of Weight Watchers' soup
cheese-slice toastie
Dinner: 'Good for You!' lasagne

Well, Day 1 of the diet and so far, so good. I'm feeling very positive and can't wait to look amazing.

Memo to me: remember this on Day 30 when I'm trying to jump out of the window.

I had a great meeting with my manager Simon Fuller today to talk about the next single, and we put in place some plans for the next month. We had been thinking about releasing another single at Christmas, but I told him I can't do anything until I lose this weight and that I'm in the depths of despair and don't know what to do. He said he'd follow it up with Nicki on Thursday.

It was interesting. He looked petrified when I told him I wanted to shed some pounds. He was terrified that people would think 19 had put me under pressure to lose weight – which, of course, they haven't.

I feel a bit in limbo. Nicki's told me to leave it with her to think about the whole thing and find me a personal trainer and dietician, but I'm desperate to get on and change things. I don't want to do this diet in public, partly because I'm not sure I can actually lose any weight. Imagine failing, like Rik Waller. He did *Celebrity Fit Club* and walked off. Everyone had been right behind him and then he went off and put on more weight – his career may never recover now.

I just want to disappear to some posh Thai resort and come back looking classy and amazing so that I can carry on with my career with everyone saying, 'Look at her! How did she do it?'

Thursday, 9 September 2004

Breakfast: nothing
Lunch: nothing
Dinner: 'Good for You!' sandwich
packet of Wotsits
bowl of tomato soup
bottle and a half of wine (as far as I can remember)

I had a fantastic meeting with Nicki today. She's still thinking about my weight loss.

I didn't eat anything properly all day, which was a bit silly really, but at least it saved me lots of calories. Yesterday was better – I had a Caesar salad with a cheese and onion toastie for lunch, and 'Good for You!' pasta and Weight Watchers' chips for dinner. In fact yesterday was great – the weather was beautiful, so I went out with my mate Trevor from Ireland, aka 'The only gay in the village'. He's staying with me because the airline he works for as a steward is based in Heathrow.

I drank water all day – and had to run to the toilet approximately 20 million times. It nearly killed me. Trevor was on my fave drink – white wine. I'm still excited and positive about this weight-loss adventure, though, and keep dreaming about the beautiful new me in a bikini.

It's nearly the weekend, so I went out tonight and had a few drinks with friends to celebrate. A load of us who grew up in together in Glasgow go away somewhere every two or three months because we've all moved apart from each other now. Tomorrow we're off to Ireland for a long weekend – can't wait.

Friday, 10 September to Monday, 13 September 2004: Weekend in Ireland

Well, I've just come back from Ireland and I'm an absolute wreck. Had a brilliant time, though. God only knows how much I've drunk over the last few days, though I was proud of myself on Friday night for refraining from getting a take-away. I have tried to be good – I ate an apple with my tea when all the girls had cake one night and I've been grilling my food instead of frying it, which is healthy, isn't it? I've even made a

WEEKEND IN IRELAND FOOD DIARY

Day 1
Breakfast: bowl of cornflakes with skimmed milk
Lunch: 2 (grilled) Quorn sausage sandwiches
Dinner: chicken tikka baguette
6 Jack Daniel's and Diet Coke

Day 2
Breakfast: 1.5 slices of brown toast
Lunch: bowl of soup
2 chicken and coleslaw sandwiches
Dinner: 3 Quorn sausages (grilled)
3 hash browns (grilled)
half a tin of Weight Watchers' beans
bottle of white wine

Day 3 *Very bad day*
Breakfast: nothing
Lunch: fried breakfast
Dinner 1: chicken
mashed potatoes
Dinner 2: 2 Quorn sausages (grilled)
2 hash browns (grilled)
slice of toast with cheese
5 Jack Daniel's and Diet Coke

Day 4 *Bad day*
Breakfast: slice of toast
bowl of soup
Lunch: large Tex Mex Burger King meal
Dinner: pepperoni pizza
bottle of white wine

real effort to do some exercise. During the day on Saturday I went out sightseeing and did a twenty-five-minute walk down a hill, which is pretty good for me – though I bussed it back, of course. And on Sunday I went for an hour-and-a-half walk along the beach. Can't believe I'm actually walking again instead of getting cabs everywhere. At this rate my love affair with the local taxi company will soon be over and my account will no longer be through the roof.

That said, I have had the odd junk-food lapse, mainly hangover-related it must be said – well, if you're out on the lash every night and not getting in till all hours in the morning, then you need something to sort yourself out the next day, don't you? And on the way back to London our flight was delayed for two hours, so by the time I got in I was so stressed out I ordered a pizza. Oh well, you can't be perfect all the time.

Thursday, 16 September 2004: London

21 stone 8 pounds

Breakfast: bowl of cornflakes with skimmed milk
Lunch: 2 sandwiches
hash brown (grilled)
Dinner: tomato pasta with jalapeño peppers
2 glasses of white wine

Back in England again after the madness of Ireland last week. The diet has been back on track for the last few days, and I'm still trying really hard until I get a personal trainer sorted out. Yesterday I had two hash browns and two Quorn sausages for breakfast – grilled, of course – a 'Good for You!' soup for lunch, and a 'Good for You!' macaroni cheese for dinner. I'm basically living off diet ready meals and Quorn sausages at the moment. Not sleeping very well because I'm so stressed about dieting. Although I think I'm doing well, I'm crap at dealing with this because I've never been unhappy with my weight before. I'm waking up every hour on the hour. All I think about at night is, 'Jesus Christ, when am I going to lose this weight?'

It's been all change at the flat too. Roxy's only seventeen and she can't really afford to stay, so she's gone back home, and my friend Laura and I have moved into a two-bed flat overlooking the river in a different part of Battersea.

I decided today that I would go to Spain for a few days, so I booked myself and Linda on the first plane tomorrow so we can go and see all our friends out there. We visit Salou in Spain regularly. Linda, or 'Loopy' – my best friend since I was fifteen – and I first went there when we were seventeen, and we had such a brilliant time that we just kept going back. We've made so many good friends there over the years.

The diet's going well, as I'm sticking to my Weight Watchers points limit, and I'll really try to be good this weekend.

Friday, 17 September to Tuesday, 21 September 2004: Holiday in Spain

Just back from another fantastic holiday in Spain, seeing all my mates who live over there. I'm seriously considering buying a house there myself.

I started off with all the right intentions as far as the diet is concerned – I knew I didn't want to weigh myself when I got home and find that I was heavier than before I left. In fact, I haven't dared go near any scales since I've been back – I'll be lucky if I haven't put on a stone. I have to keep reminding myself I put on weight ridiculously easily. It's just so hard to stick to a diet on holiday when you're out having fun every night. I'm pinning all my hopes on Simon and Nicki to fix everything now I'm back – must call Nicki to find out what's happening with the docs and the personal trainer. I just want to wave a magic wand to make this all go away!

To be honest, I'm feeling pretty down now. Why don't I have any will-power? I caught the flu on the plane back today, as usual, and now I feel like I'm dying. Losing weight is all I think about from the moment I wake up. Unless I'm drunk I just cannot deal with the knowledge of discovering what I weighed at my uncle's wedding. Was I living a lie when I thought I was happy all that time? I'm desperate. I literally just want to cut the weight off me.

One thing I'm not affected by is seeing girls in bikinis on beaches, and people are always surprised about that. The fact is that I've always been around my friends and my sisters and I'm used to it. I've always thought that the kind of guys who like those girls wouldn't go for me anyway, that I was in a different category.

Actually, I did manage to pull the most beautiful guy on the Friday night. Both of us were very drunk, but he was really fit. Got to bed in the small hours and slept till 5.30 p.m. the next day. Saw him again on the Sunday night and blanked him before he had the opportunity to do the same to me, so we didn't speak and now I feel miserable about it. It was silly, because he was really nice. I should have just gone up to him and said, 'Hi. How are you doing?'

HOLIDAY IN SPAIN FOOD DIARY

Day 1
Breakfast: chicken salad sandwich
Lunch: nothing
Dinner: Caesar salad with nachos
              14 Jack Daniel's and Diet Coke
              4 sambucas
              2 pints of lager

Day 2
Breakfast: nothing
Lunch: full Scottish breakfast
Dinner: nachos
              bottle of Budweiser
              half a pint of lager

Day 3
Breakfast: cheese and ham toastie with chips
Lunch: nothing
Dinner: melon and Parma ham
              steak with cheese sauce
              bottle of white wine
              2 Jack Daniel's and Diet Coke

Day 4
Breakfast: full English
Lunch: nothing
Dinner: chips and salad
              4 Jack Daniel's and Diet Coke
              3 sambucas

Day 5
Breakfast: sandwich
              2 hash browns (grilled)
Lunch: tomato pasta
Dinner: nachos
              bottle of white wine
              2 sambucas

Wednesday, 22 September 2004

Breakfast: nothing
Lunch: 3 Quorn sausages (grilled)
3 hash browns (grilled)
baked beans
Dinner: grilled chicken and mashed potatoes
2 glasses of white wine

Kim from the show came to stay, as we have a reunion dinner tonight with all the *Pop Idol* lot. During the show Kim and I stuck together a bit. We were both taken to Evans to shop, and the manager told us, 'Take as many clothes as you want. They're all free.' So Kim and I got a grand's worth of stuff each – free! We were showing off when we got back to the house and you could tell that the other girls were a bit put out because they were thin and gorgeous, but no one had given them any free stuff.

I'm absolutely petrified about tonight because I've obviously put on 3 stone since *Pop Idol* (when I was 18 stone) and it's the first time we've all seen each other for ages. I'm dreading it.

I've started exercising – thought I'd do 50 bicep curls with my dumbbells on each arm, 100 sit-ups and an extra 20 chest presses with the dumbbells for my bust.

At the dinner every single one of them looked at me and noticed that I'd put on weight – 3 stone is quite a lot – but the only person to say anything was Susanne, who's completely moved out of the limelight. She said, 'God, we haven't seen you for months. I thought you'd gone away and done one of those diets and were going to come back all skinny.'

Nothing could have been further from the truth. It made me really upset. Everyone thinks that because my career isn't going that great, the next thing I'm going to do is go and lose weight to try to revamp it again. And Susanne and I have a history, what with her reported comments in the press at the time of *Pop Idol*.

I went home and thought, 'I can't win. If I lose weight, people are going to think I've done it as a publicity stunt, but if I don't I'm going to go absolutely insane.'

I've just been crying my eyes out. What do I do? I'm damned if I do and damned if I don't. Either I'll be the disgusting beast who shouldn't have been allowed on television or I'll be the little girl who bowed to industry pressure.

Three a.m.: just sat bolt upright and thought, actually, stuff everyone else. I don't give a toss why other people think I'm doing this. All I know is that I'm miserable the way I am. And I can't pretend it's OK any more. It's probably the best thing Susanne could have said, because she forced me to look at things in perspective.

Thursday, 23 September 2004

Breakfast: bowl of cornflakes with skimmed milk
apple
Lunch: cheese toastie
bowl of tomato soup
apple
Dinner: pasta with vegetables
potato croquettes
Exercise: 100 sit-ups
50 bicep curls on each arm
50 leg lifts on each leg

Yesterday was a turning point for me. I had a good day on my diet. I'm totally focused now and want to lose the weight.

The Record of the Year award is coming up and I've been nominated, so I'd like to lose weight for that.

And I'm really looking forward to next week, too. Nicki has a big meeting with Channel 4 regarding a documentary that they want to do with me, which is a huge compliment. They do that kind of factual show – *Supernanny*, *How Clean is Your House?* – so well.

It's good to know you haven't been forgotten. When you've been out of the limelight for some time, you do wonder whether anyone remembers you, or if they're fed up with you. Are the public going to give two hoots?

Monday, 27 September 2004

Breakfast: bowl of cornflakes with skimmed milk
Lunch: 3 packets of cheesy Wotsits
Dinner: instant noodles and toast

It's been a pretty good weekend for sticking to the diet – I ate grilled hash browns and Quorn sausages with Weight Watchers' bread for breakfast, skipped lunch both days, and hardly had anything for dinner – a cheese toastie or nachos. I've been eating a lot of Wotsits recently, as I've discovered that – surprisingly – a 21g packet is only 2 points on the Weight Watchers system, whereas a typical lunch would be 6.

I'm starting to feel a bit better about myself, so I went to Harrods on Sunday with some friends and blew £200 on sexy underwear. Good old Rigby & Peller – making underwear for the more voluptuous lady since God knows when. I got two of the same Prima Donna set – full knickers and a bra with a flower pattern – one in chocolate brown and one in navy. I've never had any problems getting bigger underwear: Evans and Simply Be both do good ranges, and New Look used to as well.

Yesterday I went on a very healthy walk round Hyde Park with my friends and didn't eat a thing during the day. I'm really into my exercise now and loving my abs machine. And I stayed in all weekend – and didn't drink!

The Diary of a Clueless Dieter: the Verdict

So I've sussed it: losing 8 stone is all about getting as many Quorn sausages down your gullet as possible and going out on the lash four nights a week instead of five. I can't believe how easy on myself I was – using a two-hour delay at an airport as an excuse to order pizza! Obviously I was misguided there, but I'm including this because I think it is similar to many people's attempts to lose weight.

In the early days, my understanding of Weight Watchers was that you could eat whatever you wanted as long as the points added up to the right total at the end of the day. In the Weight Watchers system, each type of food is allocated a certain number of 'points' according to how calorific it is and you're given a limit of how many points you're allowed to get through every day, depending on how big you are to start with (bigger people have a higher allowance because they need a higher calorie intake just to maintain their basic resting energy levels – it takes more energy to carry all that weight around!). Now, a girl of the size I was then is allowed 30 points a day, so, in theory at least, I could eat a Big Mac (9.5 points) and chips (5 points) and leave it at that. Sorted.

Although I attended their classes, which explained the principles of healthy eating, I didn't really pay much attention. They were at the end of the day and I was tired after work. So all the stuff about how you should eat five portions of fruit and vegetable daily, how you should drink eight glasses of water, how you should have an active lifestyle and so on, just went over my head. I came away with their little booklet containing a list of all the points values, and I just looked up the value of all my usual favourite foods.

When I lost the weight while preparing for my role as a bridesmaid, I did Weight Watchers. Weight Watchers can really work, but in retrospect I can see I just got too distracted by the points system without paying enough attention to what they were telling me about how to put together a healthy diet. There are women who have lost 10 stone with Weight Watchers and then kept it off – and that's great, they're better women than I am. It wasn't the solution for me, though. I found it too easy to justify sticking to my usual routines as long as I stayed within my points 'limit' – getting the same food from the Chinese takeaway, the same curry once a week.

One good thing I found about it, though, was that it really motivates you, because you see results really quickly – it took me about two weeks to lose 8 pounds using the Weight Watchers diet. The only other diet I've tried was Scottish Slimmers when I was fifteen. They give you a list of low-calorie foods you're allowed and let you have three meals a day and four snacks. I attended classes with my Aunt Caroline over a three-month period and lost about one and a half stone in all. So these diets definitely can work. But when I tried Weight Watchers this time round I wasn't paying any attention to the nutritional values of what I was eating. I was still eating the same crap – it's just that it was crap with a lower points value. So instead of having a packet of my favourite type of crisps, Doritos (4 points), I'd have cheesy Wotsits (2 points), which might have a lower calorific value but they're still chock-full of additives, salt and other stuff you don't want in your body.

Once I went on the You Are What You Eat plan – more of which later – I learned that as a general rule it was better to eat something natural and unprocessed, even if it had a higher calorific value than the 'diet' alternative. Modern food-processing techniques destroy so many vitamins, minerals and other nutrients. So, for example, if you're going to have cheese, go for something simple like a soft white cheese, which isn't fermented or matured. It can be high in fat but it also contains lots of good calcium and B vitamins. Or choose other quality cheeses, like cheddar, that are allowed to mature naturally. Don't have a processed-cheese slice, because it's full of crap – it's just a slice of chemicals, basically. Processed cheese goes through a ridiculous number of manufacturing processes, including salting and adding of preservatives and artificial flavouring agents, slicing, packaging in plastics and so on, so that many of the nutrients that are there to start with get lost along the way. I've seen cheese slices that are made from only 6 per cent cheese – and are blended with milk proteins, vegetable oils, water and artificial flavourings and additives. And this is what we fill our children with.

I was also making the classic clueless dieter's mistake of skipping meals, thinking I was 'saving' calories. In fact, I now know that it's one of the worst things I could have done to my body. We all really need a breakfast after the 'fast' of the previous night, as the body's first need is a boost of energy to kick-start the metabolism to make it work efficiently and smoothly. The brain also needs food first thing, because it requires glucose energy to enable you to think clearly. If you miss breakfast, your concentration will suffer – you'll feel sluggish and grumpy, get headaches, suffer mood swings and you're more likely to pick at unhealthy food as a result. Bad news. More importantly if you're dieting, regular eating encourages the body to burn more fuel. Plenty of research suggests that dieters who skip meals are more likely to remain overweight than those eating three daily meals. Skipping meals regularly tricks the body into thinking that food is scarce – in other words, it triggers 'starvation mode' and as a survivalist mechanism the body begins to store fat. Which is the exact opposite of what you want if you're trying to lose weight.

I've also discovered that one study has shown that skipping meals improved the taste of sweet foods – so denying yourself all day then eating something sweet at the end of the day will make it taste so good it'll encourage you to eat more than you would normally. Fortunately, as I don't have a sweet tooth, that wasn't so much of a problem for me.

Going back to Weight Watchers, the one thing I really did like about it was going to meetings and getting weighed every week. I found it much better to go on the scales there once a week than to keep scales in my house and end up going on them every day. It's the most depressing thing in the world because if you start weighing yourself every day it will move up and down according to things like whether you've peed before weighing. And remember, the You Are What You Eat *plan is not just about losing weight – it's about overhauling your whole approach to healthy eating. So don't get obsessed about what the scales tell you.*

Involve someone – your friend or your mum. Having someone to support you if you're making a big lifestyle change really helps. And be patient. If you're eating healthily and really thinking about what you're putting in your mouth, be happy with that. The dress sizes will drop naturally, honestly. You Are What You Eat *is much more about improving your overall diet, rather than simply losing weight.*

Maybe it's to do with having an addictive personality – or no imagination – but in the old days, once I was hooked on to something I ate it all the time. Quorn sausages appear every day in my food diary at one point. I remember getting through absolutely loads of those 'Good for You!' meals because they were cheaper if you bought them in bulk. Not all diet-branded foods are bad for you, of course, but the thing to bear in mind with them is that nutritional content is not their priority. So, often, what you'll find is that these sorts of foods contain lots of artificial flavourings and sweeteners that don't carry calories, but do carry a lot of taste, which can 'spoil' the palate. If you rely on these foods all the time it's harder to enjoy the taste of real, hearty food. Once in a while, if you want a lo-cal meal, they're OK. They have their place. But I know now it's a mistake to rely on them all the time as if they're the answer to your prayers.

And crucially, I didn't realize how much alcohol contributes to weight gain. I'd always assumed that drinking was something that all normal, cool, young people did. It couldn't do any harm. Especially not a spirit like Jack Daniel's with Diet Coke. What could be healthier? What I didn't know was that alcohol provides 7 calories per gram, which may not sound a lot, but when you consider that fat is not much higher, at 9 calories per gram, you'll realize how much this is.

To put it in context, a single Jack Daniel's and Coke is 110 calories, a JD and Diet Coke is 60 calories, a medium glass of red wine is about 120 calories, and – shockingly – a double Bailey's is over 160 calories. On a big night out, it's easy to get through 1,000 calories in drink alone – half the guideline daily intake for the average woman – and that's before you count the bar snacks . . .

Booze also contains 'empty calories' – in other words, it offers little or no nutritional benefit. For example, an apple has 50 or so calories, mostly found in its natural fruit sugars. These aren't empty, because apples offer fibre, vitamin C and antioxidants. A can of Coke, on the other hand, has about 140 calories – but these are 'empty', because they contain no vitamins, no useful minerals, no fibre, no protein, no useful nutrients at all.

You can trick yourself with the effects of alcohol, too. If you get hammered the night before, you lose weight through dehydration before your body realizes what's going on. You think you've lost fat but it's just water, and of course you've put it on again by the next day. One way or another, alcohol is terrible for a dieter. It's a diuretic, which means if you drink it draws water out from all the body's cells, encouraging you to pee more, which can lead to dehydration. This, believe it or not, causes your brain to shrink away from your skull, triggering your hangover! And because you lose vital minerals when you drink, and because your blood-sugar levels are lowered when you drink (as glucose is lost in urine), the next day you'll have a taste for very salty and sugary food – hence the urge for a big fry-up.

I wasn't completely ignorant. I knew booze played a part in my weight gain, but I thought if I cut it out once or twice a week then that would be enough. In the beginning, it was never an option to cut my darling alcohol out of my life completely. Cutting back also made me feel like a martyr. Like I'd done double work. I had a ridiculous mindset back then. Why did I bother saying I was trying to lose weight if I wasn't going to commit to it?

What happened with me on this diet is pretty typical of a lot of people who try to lose weight this way without knowing what they're doing, I think. You get two or three months down the line, by which time you've lost 2 or 3 stone, and you feel fantastic. Then you're on a night out, and you've been drinking Jack Daniel's and Diet Coke, and the bar's out of Diet Coke, so you have a normal Coke. And then you stop off at the garage on the way home because you haven't eaten anything and they've got no Wotsits. So you get Doritos, thinking, 'It's not going to kill me. I've been so good this week.' And then you're right back to the beginning.

I was in desperate need of re-education. In my head I thought I was doing my body the world of good by pumping it full of alcohol, but grilling my bacon instead of frying it. Looking back, I can't believe that I was also really proud of myself for doing a twenty-five-minute walk – downhill!

As well as falling for the whole diet-food branding thing, I thought I could buy myself thin in other ways. I bought myself an ab-cruncher, an exercise bike and a step machine on the Shopping Channel. Of course, within no time the only thing I was using them for was drying clothes.

And I hardly lost any weight at all.

PHASE II – McKEITHED!

Wednesday, 29 September 2004

I found out what the 'documentary' is today.

I had a meeting with Nicki and Simon Fuller, who told me that the production company Celador – who make *Who Wants To Be A Millionaire?* – would love me to appear on *You Are What You Eat*. To be honest, I've never dared watch the show, but I've heard all about it – it's everywhere. It's always been too close to home for me – watching the holistic nutritionist Gillian McKeith tell all those overweight people what they're doing wrong made for uncomfortable viewing.

Nicki said I'd be an inspiration to all those other over-weight women who were as big as I was and who were trying to lose weight, but my first response was to say no, I don't want to do it on TV. This is huge scale for me: Channel 4; Gillian McKeith; 'celebrity special'.

Nicki said if it was her, she would do it, because doing this on TV would make her stick to the diet. She said she was only going on how desperately I'd been saying I wanted to lose weight. She also pointed out that Gillian has helped many people, and would cost a small fortune to consult privately.

I'm not sure, though. What if I fail? It's one thing to fall off a diet when no one's watching; it's another thing altogether to do it on primetime TV. How embarrassing would it be if I agree to do it and end up not losing any weight at all? Or even worse, put more on?

Thursday, 7 October 2004

I'm coming round to the idea of the documentary, and it's all because of Nicki. I trust her completely. She fought my corner on *Pop Idol* and she's still on my side.

She works for my management company and she's a businesswoman, but she's always been there to listen to me as a friend. I don't know whether I would have had the balls to consider this without her. She's dealt with it really sensitively and done all the groundwork. Simon Fuller has too, but Nicki's really applied herself to me losing weight and has got the ball rolling.

Sunday, 10 October 2004

My only worry about *You Are What You Eat* now is that because I haven't had a single out for some time and I've dropped off the radar slightly, people will see it as a *Celebrity Big Brother* or *Celebrity Fit Club* type of programme and think I'm doing it to revamp my career.

Actually, I'm a petrified twenty-four-year-old who weighs 22 stone. I really have to do something; it's downright dangerous for my health if I don't. Why should I care if people question my motives? I'm not doing it for them. And perhaps me being in the public eye will turn out to be a positive thing – if I attempt to do this in public it will make me less likely to fail. Well, that's the theory at least.

So much for disappearing off to Thailand and coming back looking amazing! Simon Fuller told me, 'You need to do this on TV,' and added that I'd be a role model for others. In fact, 19 are all saying I should do it for me. They may have an eye on the surrounding publicity, but it doesn't feel like it.

And it's not that good for my career – all that pressure and I'm not getting a penny for it!

Wednesday, 13 October 2004

I've been thinking a lot about how happy I've always said I was with myself, and wondering whether it was true, or whether I've been in denial all this time. I think deep down I was terrified to find out what weight I was. Although I was happy with the way I looked, how you feel when you're all glammed up and the cold truth of what the bathroom scales are telling you are two different things. I am lucky enough to have some lovely, flatteringly cut clothes, and there are little tricks I can use – always buy a size bigger so it doesn't cling to you. That kind of thing.

I think in retrospect I must have had a kind of reverse anorexia – I considered myself to be a whole lot slimmer than I was. It was as if I didn't really see myself when I looked in the mirror. What I saw was just normal. You can see whatever you want to in the mirror, according to your mood.

My friend Carrie could never believe that I could go out thinking I looked great when I was a size 26. She loves the fact that no matter what size I am I can look in the mirror and think I'm beautiful. It's quite strange. I've just always really had a ticket on myself.

Friday, 22 October 2004

I've done it. I've said yes to the show. What have I let myself in for?

The first indication that I might have bitten off more than I can chew was when a bizarre package arrived in the post a few days ago. Apparently, I have to send my poo to America to have it analysed! There were full instructions in the parcel. I had to poo into this basin. Enclosed was a test tube full of acid, which had a lid with a scooper attached. I had to scoop the best part of the poo (!) into this test tube, then mash it all together in the acid. Last of all I had to give it a good shake until there were no more poo particles and it was a nice brown liquid. When it's your own, it's not so bad. If it was someone else's, I'd have passed out.

MICHELLE'S GUIDE TO POO

Big Poo

Small Poo

Smelly Poo

Hangover Poo

Upset tummy – bicycle clips
needed to prevent leakage

I had to do that for four days. I left the collection of samples in the bottom of the bathroom cupboard. Laura said if I brought them out of the cupboard she was leaving. Perhaps I should have borrowed one of her poos to see if they noticed the difference.

It's probably just someone at Celador having a laugh, or maybe Gillian gets her kicks by being a poo collector. I've not seen the show before, but I'm told they always analyse the poor victim's poo each week. Apparently you can tell a lot about your health according to what your waste looks like.

Thursday, 4 November 2004

Today I meet the famous Gillian McKeith – but before I do, Nicki is going to explain to me what *You Are What You Eat* is all about.

It's not about dieting, apparently, but about making a 'long-term lifestyle change'. The people behind it don't think traditional weight-loss plans and trendy fad diets work or are very good for you, because they deprive you of things your body needs. The production company says it's aimed at people desperate for information on how to make healthy decisions. They started off thinking that the subject might be of interest to enough people to make a television programme, but then they realized how big the demand was when *You Are What You Eat* became a huge global brand. It took them by surprise that there should be such a demand for something so simple. It makes you realize how many people – like me – genuinely don't know much about how to eat healthily and are crying out for more reliable information. We're bombarded with advertising from the food industry about the latest 'lite' or 'low-fat' food, and stories from celebrities who reckon they've achieved miracles on some crazy fad diet, but back in the real world it can be difficult to work out what's genuinely good for you and worth putting in your supermarket trolley, and what's best avoided. Without an understanding of the basics of a healthy diet, how can we make good choices about which foods to put in our bodies?

The emphasis on the *You Are What You Eat* plan is to stop and think before you eat or drink anything, so that you take responsibility for yourself. Blimey. What sounds good about it is that you can eat as much as you like of the right things. If you have a punnet full of blueberries for breakfast, but you're still hungry, have another, Gillian says.

On an average show, they take someone who's pretty unhealthy and typically very overweight, and they send in Gillian McKeith to look at his or her diet and assess what needs changing. (Normally, it's pretty much everything.) They then follow that person's progress, as he or she tries to stick to the new rules over the course of eight weeks, and at the end they look at how much better the person feels, after the benefits of the new natural diet have really kicked in. The results are generally pretty dramatic, and the volunteers always say they'll carry on with the regime now they under-stand how it works. People tend to lose weight on this plan, but that's not the main emphasis – *You Are What You Eat* reckon it's more important to eat healthily than simply to focus on dropping a dress size. Obviously in my case, though, we do need to shift some serious excess pounds – apparently, most people who go on the show aren't as overweight in rela-tion to their height as I am. Great.

As a result, I'm going to be following this plan for a whole year – gulp – and I'll be getting support from both the show itself and Gillian. The idea is that I'll be introduced to the main principles of the *You Are What You Eat* diet for life, which will start re-educating me about food, then I'll have daily back-up from Gillian in the form of regular meetings, phone calls, text messages, recipe suggestions etc. The idea is that this will keep me motivated. Apparently, Gillian is a brilliant motivator.

All the girls in the 19 office have bought the *You Are What You Eat* book in preparation for Gillian's visit. They've stocked up the cupboards with peppermint tea and nettle tea, and binned all the coffee and fizzy drinks. This is what the threat of this woman's presence does to people. She has these girls in an absolute tizzy.

I'm sitting in the office thinking, 'Who is this woman? Everyone's petrified of her.'

In preparation for the big meeting, I was given a massive questionnaire to fill out: everything from what I'd had for breakfast to what colour my poos were and how they flowed. (I swear they're poo perverts, these people.) It also covered my family's health. Is there obesity in the family? No. How much exercise do I do? Almost none. Do I get out of breath? Well, it depends what I'm doing, doesn't it? Do I have any allergies/skin conditions? None. Do I snore? You could say that – it's almost ruined relationships.

There were more bizarre questions, too. What colour were my eyes? Did I have spots on my tongue? My initial impression of this woman before meeting her is that she's completely batty. I'm intrigued to see what she's like in person. I'm sure this degree of detail isn't necessary for people starting to lose weight, but I suppose it's good to take a long hard look at yourself.

Eventually, in trots this very slim lady with her nose stuck in the air. She glances over at me and then sits at Simon

Fuller's desk. Then, without making eye contact, she starts flicking through the questionnaire.

'You have *how* many units of alcohol on a Friday night?'

'Well, what night are you looking at? What does it say?'

'It tells me here you had eight Jack Daniel's in one night.'

'Oh that must have been a Wednesday or a Thursday. That wasn't the weekend.'

All this time, Nicki was looking daggers at me, as if to say, 'Do *not* wind her up because she hasn't agreed to do this show yet.'

Then Gillian asked me all these questions about my poo in front of the whole room. I thought, 'You're not going to embarrass me, love. I'll just tell you about it.'

'Gillian, it smells like shit, what does yours smell like?'

She just looked at me.

'It's called shit for a reason,' I went on. 'Your body rejects it. It's not supposed to smell like a rose.' She was really getting on my nerves and putting on the whole I'm Going to Eat You Alive persona – wrong choice of phrase, because she wouldn't eat anything my size.

At the end of the meeting she said, 'Right, OK. Well, we'll be in touch.' And she walked out.

I looked at the girls in the office, and asked them, 'What does that mean? Does she want to work with me or what? What's happening?'

'I think she really liked you,' said Nicki.

Monday, 8 November 2004

Today I met Damon Pattison and Claire Masters from Celador at Ransome's Dock in London. 'Gillian's up for it,' they told me, 'let's do this TV show.'

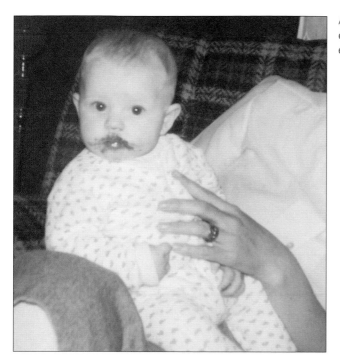

Aged six months, enjoying my first ever chocolate bar.

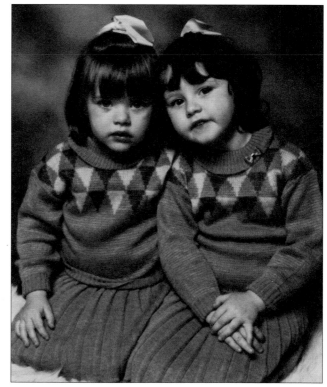

With my sister Lynsey (*left*), at age three. I didn't start life as a large child: I was a healthy, normal size as a young girl.

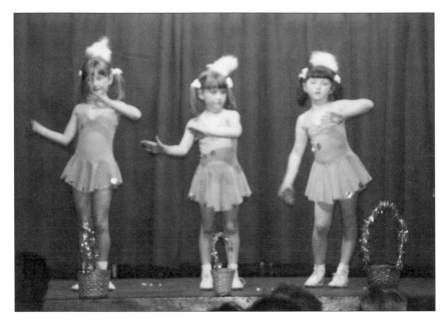

Michelle McManus the ballet dancer! (*right*) I never lost my passion for performing, but the leotards and regular exercise soon went by the wayside.

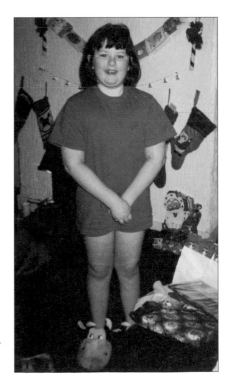

Christmas Day 1990. The weight is starting to creep on.

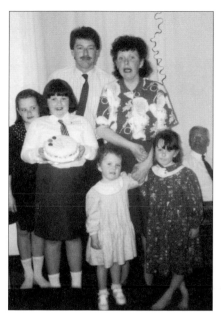

With my family, aged ten, at my first confirmation. My family have been nothing but supportive of me all my life. Note Dad's dodgy moustache!

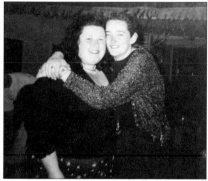

Aged nineteen on holiday, with my good pal Linda.

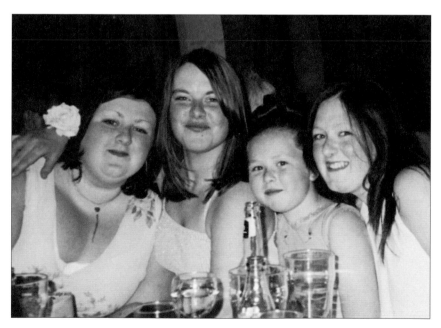

WE ARE FAMILY: From l-r with sisters Lynsey, Kerry and Laura at our uncle's wedding in 2001. None of my family is overweight, but I've never been jealous of their slim figures – I always reasoned that everyone is different.

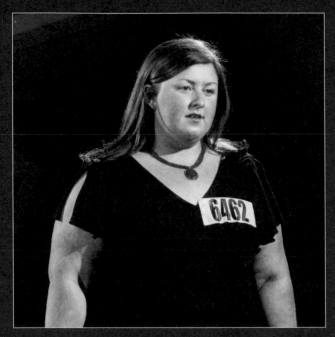

My first audition for *Pop Idol* in May 2003. I could sense straightaway that the judges were thinking, 'What is this girl thinking of?'

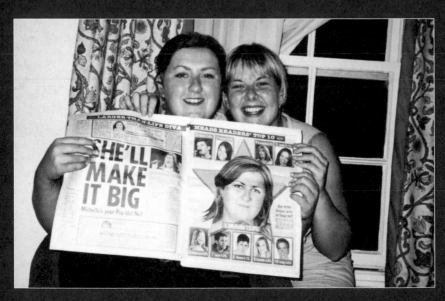

Lynsey and I celebrating my first time in the papers, once I'd made it to the final fifty. I was so thrilled it was a positive piece; I'd feared I was going to be slaughtered for being overweight. The respite, of course, proved short-lived.

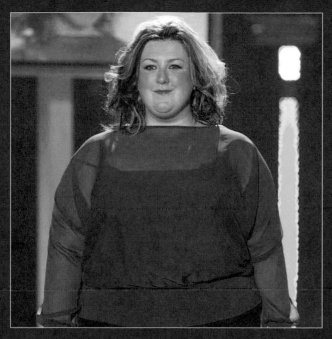

SHE'S A STAR: Performing on *Pop Idol*. The stylists managed to wean me from my favourite all-black outfits: it wasn't always a successful move.

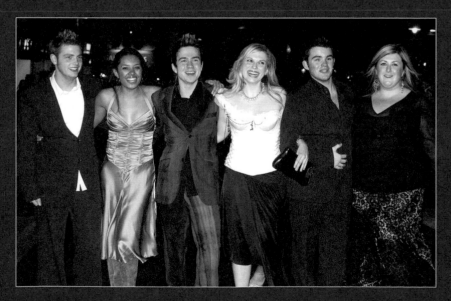

With the gang at the film premiere of *Love Actually*, feeling like a proper celebrity! Joining me on the red carpet, from l-r: fellow finalist Mark Rhodes, good mate Roxanne, bookies' favourite Sam Nixon, Susanne Manning and Chris 'the vicar' Hyde.

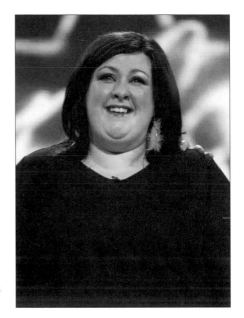

WILL I STAY OR WILL I GO?: The moment of elimination. My nerves were always awful, even though, once Kim left, my fear that the public were just keeping me in because I was big was put to rest.

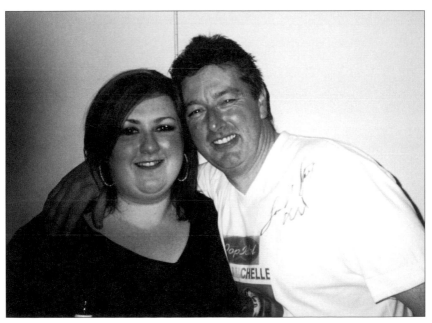

Just got through to the final! With proud dad.

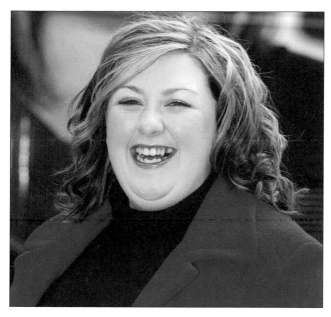

Out and about on the campaign trail. At a photo call (*left*) and with my *Pop Idol* battle bus (*below*).

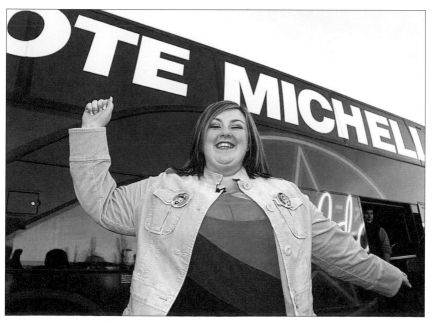

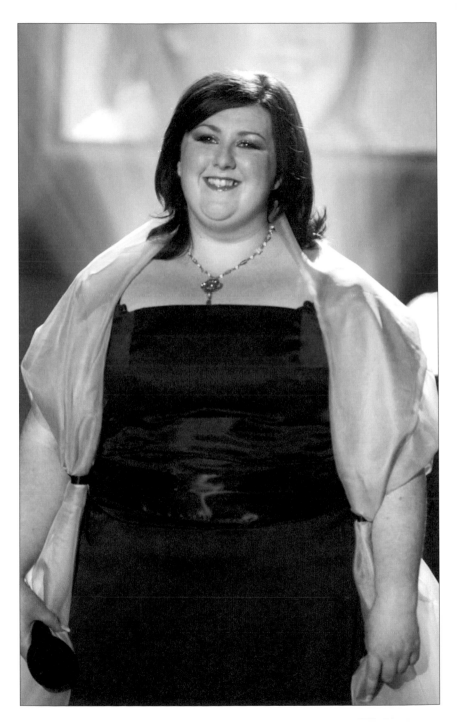

The moment I never thought would come: winning *Pop Idol*. How I did it wearing 'that dress', I'll never know.

But there was 'a problem'. The *You Are What You Eat* plan always starts with an eight-week detox, which means I'd be having to eat a fairly restricted diet for those weeks, before gradually reintroducing other foods. And as they explained, 'We have to start with Gillian on 4 December, which means you'd be doing the detox over Christmas. How do you feel about that?'

I can read TV people like a book these days. They were loving the fact that I was going to be detoxing over Christmas, because of course this meant Jeopardy Scenario No. 1. 'Jeopardy' is a reality-TV concept that I learned about at *Pop Idol*. It's like when they wheel in a six-foot blonde on *Big Brother* when there's already a couple in there starting a relationship, just to try to bust them up. If two favourites were up for being voted off in the same week on *Pop Idol*, that was jeopardy.

I told them that was fine, I'd manage it over Christmas. I can't tell you how impatient I am to get started. It's a combination of waiting since September, failing miserably at this pathetic diet I've been on with the Quorn sausages – I'm back up to 22 stone – and meeting Gillian and wanting to prove her wrong.

I'm getting to a stage where I really can't take carrying this weight around any more. I'm not even stabilizing, I'm up and down 4 pounds either way the whole time. I've had enough.

I've started to look at some of the *You Are What You Eat* information that they left me with. The good news is that there's lots of things that I can eat on this diet. Oh, and I really must remember not to call it a 'diet' – it's a 'plan'. *You Are What You Eat* don't believe in dieting as such – they say you can eat as much as you want if you stick to the right 'good' food choices. You should never go hungry as the portions of these foods aren't restricted.

YOU ARE WHAT YOU EAT 'GOOD' FOODS I'VE HEARD OF

Fruit
All dried fruit
Apples
Apricots
Avocados
Bananas
Blackberries
Blueberries
Cherries
Cranberries
Currants
Dates
Figs
Gooseberries
Grapefruit
Grapes
Kiwi fruits
Lemons
Limes
Mangoes
Melons
Nectarines
Oranges
Passion fruits
Peaches
Pears
Pineapples
Strawberries
Tangerines
And tomato – ha!
You can't catch
me out

Herbal teas

Herbs (fresh)

Fish

Grains
Barley
Basmati rice
Brown rice
Bulgur wheat
Corn
Oats
Quinoa

Nuts
Almonds
Brazil nuts
Cashews
Hazelnuts
Chestnuts
Pecans
Pine nuts
Pistachios
Walnuts

Pulses
Aduki
Fava
Lentils
Lima
Pinto
Soybeans

Seeds
Pumpkin
Sesame
Sunflower

Tofu

Vegetables
Artichokes
Asparagus
Aubergines
Beetroot
Broccoli
Brussels sprouts
Bok choy
Cabbages
Carrots
Cauliflower
Celery
Courgettes
Kale
Lettuce
Onions
Parsnips
Peas
Peppers
Radish
Rocket
Seaweed
Spinach
Sweet potatoes
Squash
Turnips
Watercress

**Wholewheat
breads, pasta etc.**

Friday, 12 November 2004

I've been reading more *You Are What You Eat* information. If the fact that you can eat as much as you want on this plan is the good news (though I'm not sure eating as many Brussels sprouts as I want really qualifies as being good), then here's the bad news. Every single one of the bad dishes they tell you to steer clear of in Gillian's *You Are What You Eat* book is an old friend. Chips, pizza, burgers, chicken tikka masala, Chinese takeaways, toast made with white bread, you name it. This is not going to be easy! In the book, the worst culprits are broken down to show the typical amount of fat and sugar that they each contain, and this is then converted into lard and teaspoons of sugar to give a handy visual image. It's not comfortable reading. In fact, it turned my stomach.

'Do you really still feel hungry?' it asks.

No, not really.

Tuesday, 16 November 2004

I've met with the *You Are What You Eat* crew: Ita the director, Toby the cameraman – who's gorgeous – and Phil the sound guy. Now we're setting about putting some kind of filming schedule into place.

Thursday, 18 November 2004

This poo business won't leave me alone. I've had to turn my bathroom into a makeshift poo-collection lab. This time I have to do a poo, catch it in a net and put it in a container for Gillian. Then some poor bastard has to come over and collect it.

Apparently, you have to be careful not to base all your analysis on just one poo as they change according to our previous day's diet and other factors such as stress levels and fluid intake. So if you're going to start checking them out, you have to do it regularly.

THE LOWDOWN ON POO

Some nutritionists use poo analysis to help them assess the condition of your health and diet. Below are some of the things your poo may say about you, but always consult your doctor if anything worries you about your poo, rather than relying solely on self-diagnosis.

If your poo:

. . . is greasy/fatty and it floats, or is light-coloured, then this could signify a liver problem and/or fat-digestion problem. This could have many causes. Your diet could be low in cruciferous green vegetables (like cabbage, cauliflower and broccoli, for instance). Alternatively, you may be eating a diet too high in fat, and your liver, which produces the enzymes that digest fat in the body, may not be able to cope with the volume. Eating more omega-3 fatty acids, found in oily fish, nuts and seeds, can help.

. . . stinks to high heaven, then this can signify over-fermentation of your food in the bowel, probably because your intestinal transit (the time taken between eating a food and passing its waste out) is too long, typically over forty-eight hours. Slow intestinal transit is caused by a diet low in fruit and vegetables, and high in processed foods and simple starchy carbohydrates.

. . . contains bits of undigested food, then you could be rushing your eating, and not chewing it enough. It's also possible that your digestive system is weak, again as a result of a poor diet. You'll need to make a point of eating more slowly: as Gillian says, 'Your stomach doesn't have any teeth.' Which is an attractive image, no?

. . . looks like any of the following: hard, pellet-like stools, excessively runny stools, mushy stools that stick to the side of the bowl or require you to wipe a lot – these can all be signs that your diet needs improving, though it's difficult to diagnose specific problems as there could be lots of causes. See your doc if you're worried. Likewise, if you spot any worms in there.

. . . contains blood, don't panic. It sounds horribly serious, but may not be. It could be simply haemorrhoids (piles), although at the other end of the scale it could be an early-warning sign of bowel cancer. Get it checked out immediately, just in case. Vigorous wiping of your bum can cause skin to tear and bleed, so don't be alarmed if you see bright red blood on the loo paper when you wipe – just go easy on the Andrex in future, OK?

. . . displays any other unusual characteristics. For example, if you have diarrhoea or constipation, either separately or alternating, then it might be a sign of irritable bowel syndrome or other digestive conditions such as food intolerances. Likewise, if there's a drastic change in frequency. In both cases, a little visit to your doc's would be recommended.

Friday, 19 November 2004

I went to Glasgow to see the family and get thoroughly checked out by the doctor prior to starting *You Are What You Eat*. He said there was nothing wrong with me apart from the fact that

I'm 'morbidly obese'. What a lovely phrase. The blood-test results are still to come, but he expects them all to be clear.

I haven't told any of my family yet what I'm about to do. It's really unnatural being so secretive with everybody, but I know what my sisters will be like if I tell them I'm making a serious attempt to lose weight. They'll say I don't need to and that they all love me the way I am.

I think we're all pretty reluctant to embrace change. It reminds me of Dad's moustache when we were little – we wouldn't let him get rid of it, even though it wasn't in fashion. No one had a moustache and he had to go through the whole of the Nineties with an Eighties' moustache because we wouldn't let him shave it off. When he actually did it once, we all screamed the house down.

Of course, he hasn't got a moustache now and he looks about twenty-five years younger.

Monday, 22 November 2004

I'm back in London – my friends are helping me to say a final emotional farewell to junk food and booze. We went for pizza tonight. Mine was a pepperoni washed down with a bottle or so of white wine. Farewell, flab.

Wednesday, 24 November 2004

I realized I haven't quite said all my goodbyes. Tonight, I jumped into a family pack of Doritos – *'You're* my family' – and a bottle of Chablis.

Thursday, 25 November

Friends June, Laura and Linda came round to visit and we watched *Pride and Prejudice* while eating curry and drinking champagne. Surely there's no harm in building up my strength for filming?

Monday, 29 November 2004

I've been having a few meetings with Gillian over the past few days. She's psyching me up for my initial detox and explaining how my life has to change. She keeps sitting me down and talking me through healthy eating and losing weight. She's made me realize that what a lot of people do – myself included – is just turn straight to the back of food packets and look only at the calorie content. If they read that something contains fewer than 300 calories, they think it's a good healthy meal, whereas what they should really be looking at is the ingredients.

If you buy a tuna salad, what should be in that salad? Tuna, lettuce, tomato, onion, dressing. Nothing else. But if you look at the back of a typical pre-packed tuna salad, you'll see it's got preservatives like sulphur dioxide, E numbers, MSG (which contains sodium) – all sorts of rubbish. Now I've started to look, I can't believe the number of ingredients in these things, and there's always way too much salt. Salt soaks up all the liquid in your body, resulting in water retention – it's basically your body's attempt to dilute the salt in your system. It can add several pounds to your body weight. Too much salt raises your blood pressure, which of course has a knock-on effect on your heart (which is made to work harder) and your arteries (which have to deal with greater strains). It means you'll feel sluggish and bloated as a result of the extra weight (of water) you're carrying and the tiredness caused by a harder-working heart. I've now learned that, mad as it sounds, you need to drink more water if you're suffering from water retention, to flush out the salt.

So it's the ingredients, not just the calorie content, that people should be looking at. Gillian says you should be cautious about any ingredient name you don't recognize.

We also discussed some of the important rules I'm going to be living by from now on. I call them 'The Rules', or 'The Ten Commandments'.

THE RULES

I. NO WHITE BREAD/RICE/PASTA OR POTATOES – CHOOSE WHOLEGRAIN OR WHOLEMEAL CARBS INSTEAD

In other words, no refined carbohydrates – food made from refined grains such as refined wheat and white rice. Refined grains have been stripped of their outer coating, their bran and their germ (i.e. wheatgerm) during processing, leaving only what's called the endosperm. It's the endosperm that is ground into flour and made into bread or pasta. Because a large proportion of the nutrients in the original grain (90 per cent) is contained in the germ and bran, there's very little of nutritional value left in this flour and in the products made with it. To compensate, white bread flour is fortified with B vitamins, calcium and iron in the UK, but the body is not able to absorb these added nutrients as efficiently as if they were found naturally within the food.

Wholegrain or wholemeal products, on the other hand – for example, brown bread and brown pasta – are made from grains that aren't stripped of their goodness and are more filling and nutritious. They're a much better food choice.

The other problem with refined grains is that the carbs they contain are very easily and quickly digested by the body. This can cause the blood glucose levels to rise sharply and then dip just as sharply after a short period, leading to hunger pangs as soon as an hour after you've eaten. With wholegrain food, however, the body has to work harder to digest it. Slower digestion means slower absorption of the food, leading to a slow and gradual rise in blood glucose levels, which keeps hunger at bay for much longer.

It's only a rough rule, but white food is usually the less healthy option. Always go for the darker option. Brown bread is better than white bread. Brown rice is better than white rice. Whole pot barley is better than white pearl barley, and so on.

As for potatoes, they are one of the starchiest vegetables. They're not bad for you as such – they're one of the highest sources of vitamin C in a typical British diet, and they contain several B vitamins and the mineral potassium, which is useful in regulating blood pressure. They're also virtually fat free. However, because they're so 'easy' to eat – and to overeat – the *You Are What You Eat* plan encourages you to experiment with other vegetables that you may not normally consider consuming. Also, potatoes don't count towards your government-recommended five portions of fruit and veg a day.

If you miss the potato's texture and sweetness, try sweet potatoes – which are allowed, as they're not related to the potato. They're a fantastic substitute and rich in antioxidants such as betacarotene. They're delicious roasted, boiled or mashed.

2. NO ADDED SALT

Eighty-five per cent of men and 69 per cent of women eat too much salt – a habit that raises your blood pressure and triples your risk of heart disease and stroke. Adults should not consume more than 6g of salt daily – roughly one teaspoonful.

Three-quarters of the salt we eat is found as an ingredient in prepared foods, but it's not always simple to identify which foods are high or low in salt. As a rough guideline, less than 0.25g of salt per 100g of overall product is deemed as a 'little' amount of salt, between 0.25g and 1.25g per 100g is a 'moderate' amount, and anything over 1.25g per 100g is 'a lot'. (Note that salt is sometimes expressed as sodium on labelling. To calculate the salt content from the sodium content, multiply the sodium value by 2.5. So 1g of sodium actually equals 2.5g of salt – a very high amount.)

A small 40g bag of Doritos, for example, contains close to 1g of salt (as well as 200 calories), so you can see how easy it is to go over the 6g daily amount.

Because it's so easy to consume more than the recommended 6g, it's important not to add more salt to foods you prepare yourself. Always taste food first that you would normally sprinkle with salt – only very rarely does food need seasoning, and if you feel it does need extra flavour, experiment instead with pepper or fresh herbs.

Typical foods low in salt are fruit, vegetables, sweets, honey and nuts.

Typical foods with medium salt content are meats, yoghurt, milk, eggs and fish.

Typical food with high salt content are processed meats, cheese and smoked fish.

3. AVOID PRE-PACKAGED AND PROCESSED FOODS, E.G. MICROWAVE MEALS, PACKET SANDWICHES ETC.

Processed ready meals and pre-prepared snacks tend to contain a great deal of artificial flavourings, additives and preservatives, so it's good to try to avoid over-relying on these if you're aiming for a healthy, natural diet. Making meals from scratch forces you to use fresh ingredients and really think about what you're putting into your body. If you're making your own pasta sauce, for example, you'd never put in as much salt as what the average jar of pre-prepared sauce contains. Eating pre-prepared food gets you into the habit of eating thoughtlessly. Also, preparing your own food stimulates your digestive juices, so when you do eat the meal, your body is ready to receive it. And making your own food means you can keep portion sizes under control.

4. AVOID MIXING CARBS AND PROTEIN

As your body metabolizes your food, the proteins you eat need acidic digestive juices and the carbohydrates need alkaline digestive juices in order for the body to be able to utilize them properly. It's believed that eating proteins and carbohydrates together can cause the differing classes of enzyme to 'compete' and neutralize one another, leading to the inefficient digestion of both carbs and proteins – which can cause wind, bloating, heartburn, indigestion and sluggishness.

Vegetables can be eaten either with proteins (such as meats) or with carbohydrates (such as grains), but proteins and carbs together (for instance, a meaty rice dish or pasta with a bolognese sauce) should be avoided. Fruit is a separate case: it should always be eaten separately, at least half an hour before or after any other food or meal (see Rule Number 8).

5. CUT OUT ALCOHOL COMPLETELY FOR THE FIRST EIGHT WEEKS AND DRINK IN MODERATION THEREAFTER

There are lots of reasons to avoid the demon drink if you're trying to eat healthily. By and large, it contains 'empty' calories (see page 54); it dehydrates your body severely; it's addictive; and from a dieting viewpoint, it can both weaken your resolve when you're under the influence and also lead to cravings for salty or sugary foods the next day.

Certainly, your internal organs will thank you if you cut out alcohol. Booze overloads and overworks the liver's several hundred functions. Many of these functions are to do with digestion: if you 'bother' the liver with added work by giving it a lot of alcohol to detoxify, it can't get on with the much more important jobs in the body, like digestion of fats. Give your liver a break!

Alcohol also puts increased strain on the heart and cardio-vascular system, because it forces the blood vessels to constrict, compelling the heart to work harder to get oxygen to your body's cells. If you're overweight, your heart is likely to be already working much harder than it ought to, so it certainly doesn't need the additional stress and exertion. So give your heart a break too!

One of the things people don't tend to talk about regarding alcohol is that in the longer term, those who drink frequently tend to be more depressed and miserable. From a dieter's perspective, this can lead to seeking 'refuge' in comfort food, which in turn can result in a skewed relationship with eating.

6. CUT OUT CAFFEINE COMPLETELY FOR THE FIRST EIGHT WEEKS AND DRINK IN MODERATION THEREAFTER

Caffeine is a stimulant drug most famously found in coffee, although it's also present in more moderate amounts in tea (black, green and white), cola drinks, chocolate, and in some painkilling tablets.

The bad press caffeine gets isn't entirely justified – in moderation, it's an excellent mental energizer and mood lifter; it can relieve asthmatic symptoms; and it's a mild painkiller (hence its use in painkilling tablets).

However, it is moderately addictive, and worse, it can induce a string of unpleasant short-term symptoms in those sensitive to it, including nausea, anxiety and agitation, tremors, mood swings, restlessness, an uneven heartbeat, vertigo, headaches, sweats and sleep interruption. More menacing reactions such as hyperventilation, panic attacks, migraines, vomiting, abdominal cramps and diarrhoea are not uncommon at higher doses. Long-term, it can be the cause of some cases of constipation.

On balance, and because coffee doesn't provide any essential nutrients, giving up caffeine for a while is a good thing to try – not least because it'll force you to experiment with other drinks such as tasty gentle herbal teas and freshly squeezed juices. Of course, you will also need to drink more water instead, which can help to flush out the system.

7. TRY TO WALK EVERYWHERE

It's simple common sense: reclaim walking as the easy way to incorporate exercise into your daily life. Walking is one of the most effective forms of exercise because it carries no risk. Whereas joggers risk knee or ankle strains, tennis players are prone to tennis elbow, and footballers sustain all manner of nasty knocks, walkers are smug in their injury-free state. A lot of people who want to lose weight think they need to join a gym or 'punish' themselves in order to get to a healthy weight – 'no pain, no gain' is their maxim – but this is unrealistic for many people, and isn't necessarily healthy. According to many health and wellbeing experts, it's more important to incorporate enjoyable *activities* into your daily life, rather than doing exercises you hate. For instance, walking to and from your amateur dramatics class, which you love, is far better than driving to the gym and doing thirty minutes of cycling or running-machine work that you absolutely hate.

8. LEAVE AT LEAST A THIRTY-MINUTE GAP AFTER EATING FRUIT AND BEFORE EATING ANYTHING ELSE

Eating fresh fruit is one of the best things you can do for your body, as all fruits are rich in vitamins and many are high in antioxidants, especially if you eat them uncooked. (Remember, it's important to aim for at least five portions of fruit and vegetables daily.) However, as fruit is quite rapidly digested, it makes sense to eat it on its own: if you eat it immediately after other foods (which are all digested more slowly), the fruit has nowhere to go in the digestive system – it gets 'stuck' behind other food, and will ferment in the gut, leading to all manner of digestive problems, such as wind, bloating and smelly poos.

9. START EACH DAY WITH A CUP OF HOT WATER AND LEMON

We lose around half a pound of water every night – through sweat and in breath – so having a refreshing drink to replace lost fluid first thing is an excellent way to start the day. A cup of hot water with freshly squeezed lemon will jump-start your liver and clean out your bowels from the day before, and it's a much gentler alternative to the usual caffeine-laden tea or coffee. But don't forget to have a rounded breakfast too!

10. DRINK AT LEAST 2 LITRES OF WATER DAILY

Nearly 40 per cent of us don't drink enough fluids – we all need water to replace fluids lost through sweat and going to the loo. If you don't drink enough, your digestion will suffer and you'll soon get dehydrated, which can affect your metabolism – bad news for dieters. For someone trying to lose weight, it's a useful tip to drink a glass of water instead when you start feeling like you want to pick at something, as it's very easy to confuse feelings of thirst with those of hunger.

All fluids count towards your 2-litres-a-day target – juices, squashes, even coffee and tea (though not alcohol!) – but in the first eight-week detox of the *You Are What You Eat* plan, stick to still water, preferably mineral or filtered. If you are not used to drinking large quantities of fluids, you should build up to the 2-litre level over a few days so that your body gets accustomed to dealing with the increased amounts.

Filming begins. These first couple of days are to show my backstory: the old Michelle. Me going to the nail bar and getting my nails done; me eating a pizza with Laura on the sofa; me getting taxis everywhere.

Everything was going fine. Then they said, 'Now all we need is to film you in your swimsuit.'

Toby the gorgeous cameraman does, you mean. Gulp.

'OK.'

They set up a white backdrop in my living room.

I really fancy Toby, and there he was, lying on the ground with the camera on the floor so he could get an up-shot of my thighs and my stomach. I just couldn't deal with it, because I'm feeling so low about my weight for the first time in my life. I'm not saying that I was doing cartwheels across the room when I'd been with guys before, but I was never really that self-conscious. So I was hating this new feeling and hating the fact that this gorgeous guy was going to be filming right into my thighs and my stomach.

He was really sweet, actually. He could see how upset I was because there were tears running down my face. He felt awful and even offered to strip down to his boxer shorts so that he was almost naked too. I thought, 'Mate, I fancy you. You can't be naked near me. Don't do that in my house. Then I'll be crying because you're so gorgeous.' I said, 'No – you're the sweetest man alive, but you can't strip off.'

It was Toby's job to film me in an unflattering light. He was focusing on finding the cellulite on my thighs. He didn't have to look very hard.

I don't know how people go through years and years of being unhappy with themselves, because I can't handle it at all.

The three months waiting to start the healthy-eating plan were hard enough. I kept being advised not to try to lose weight during that time and so I treated those weeks as if I had been told 'Eat as much as you can now because your life is going to be over at the end of this.' The result is that I look the worst I ever have in my life.

What nobody knows is that I wore a bodice under my swimsuit for that filming – otherwise, I would have looked even worse.

I just couldn't cope. When they left I was such a mess. I ended the day in floods of tears. I've never hated myself before. I've never felt ashamed.

What have I done? What have I let myself in for here? I don't know if I can take this. I genuinely loved myself before and now I'm putting myself through hell.

This evening I got very drunk.

Thursday, 2 December 2004

Another horrible day. Gillian came over and was completely brutal.

She started by showing me the 'good food' table and the 'bad food' table. They do this on every *You Are What You Eat* show, apparently – it's when they make you keep a food diary of what you ate over the previous week and then they make a display of all the crap you've eaten on one table to show you how bad your choices are nutritionally. Of course, it looks horrendous because it's all bacon and chips and hamburgers and so on – hardly anything green at all. Then they show you another table, which contains all the food that you're going to be eating once you're on the plan – all lovely fresh fruit and veg and wholegrains and stuff. Although I'm not normally a big fan of vegetables, it genuinely looked delicious, because I've come round to the fact that this is what I'm going to be eating from now on. Also, compared to my bad food table – which, of course, they put no presentation or effort into whatsoever; the food's cooked and left for five hours so that it's all congealed and then just chucked on paper plates – the good food table looked amazing, with all this beautifully arranged, freshly picked fruit and veg in loads of different colours.

There was my new life on the table and it was quite exciting. I have a feeling that Gillian is starting to like me now, although she absolutely laid into me about the bad food table, of course. None of it really offended me because what she was saying was true. You can't have it both ways. You can't ask for someone's help and then argue with them when they give it to you. I'm so desperate to lose weight that I was really upbeat about it all.

It's difficult to get used to the cameras being around – although they weren't filming me in a swimsuit today, thank God – and having a crew in my home. They've offered to have the carpets cleaned. Good thing too. And the rate they get through toilet paper! When it's just me and Laura, a pack of twelve rolls will get us through the month – but not when there are twenty-five people in the house. Every five minutes the cry goes up, 'We're out of toilet roll again!'

Another of Gillian's stranger habits is to lie you on the carpet and squeeze your stomach. With most people there's pain and she can say, 'Yes, that's gas right there. That means you're really unhealthy.' But I had no pain at all. She was practically doing WWF wrestling moves on me and I was fine. So she stood up, all hot and bothered, saying, 'Well, I just don't understand that. I don't know how you can be that healthy at that weight.'

She also tried to check my nails, because I think she wanted to tell me about my calcium deficiencies, but mine are acrylic and painted, which meant she couldn't get a good look at them. Ha!

HOW TO CHECK YOUR NAILS

Nails should be strong, pink, even and smooth. Healthy nails – just like healthy skin, healthy hair and so on – are more likely if you have a good diet: it's only natural that eating the right nutrients will be reflected in all aspects of your body, both internal and external. B vitamins, calcium, iron and zinc are the most important nutrients for healthy nails, but the most essential thing is a good balanced diet.

If you have any of the following problems, it's worth exploring whether you have any nutritional deficiencies, though of course there may be alternative causes, so if you're not sure, consult your doctor:

- White spots are usually caused by a minor bump to the nail. Some practitioners believe white spots – and 'ridges', or uneven nails – can be a sign of a calcium deficiency. In the case of white spots, it could indicate a zinc deficiency. Zinc is found in eggs, dairy produce and nuts.
- Splitting of nails could be a sign of low iron and zinc.
- Chronic problems with nails – such as fungal nail infections, nails that are weakly attached to the finger, and brittle nails – should be referred to a doctor, as there could be a non-nutritional cause.

On my balcony in daylight Gillian checked my tongue, which I found bizarre. Basically it showed that I was in a pretty bad way and it was a good thing that she had come along. Apparently Chinese and Eastern medicine uses tongue diagnosis widely, though I've never heard of it before. For example, a burning sensation in the tongue and/or a very smooth tongue could be a sign of iron deficiency, but, as always, contact your doctor if you have any worries.

Gillian said one horrendous thing too. 'Michelle, if you were to die tomorrow, let's hope they don't cremate you, because with the amount of alcohol in your body you'd be burning for weeks.'

What a thing to say to someone.

But the worst bit was when she presented me with eleven-and-a-half stone of animal fat to show me the equivalent of my excess weight in fat. It was just horrendous. I refused to cry on camera – I tried to take it as best I could. In a way, perhaps I should have cried. It would have made me look more human. I think it was that moment when I realized what I'd done to myself and how badly I'd abused my body. For someone who's always said they love themselves and had such a great life, I've actually been my own worst enemy. Gillian said that I had more chance of throwing a six on a dice than of living to what should be my life expectancy. She didn't elaborate. She didn't need to. She just said I'd die young if I didn't sort myself out. To let my body get into this state at twenty-four years old is just not acceptable.

Maybe I'm too controlling, but I was upset that the TV crew hadn't pre-warned me about that bit – though I suppose they wouldn't, because they wanted to see my reaction. I lost a bit of confidence in them for that. The crew felt like mates by then and I was humiliated in front of everyone. I'd forgotten that they were there to do a job and make a TV show. I told them, 'I understand what you've done today but

I think you've been out of order.' I know everyone cheats on TV shows a bit, but I just wish they'd given me a quick heads up that something not nice was about to come up. Anything. Maybe they'd forgotten that I hadn't watched the show before, so I didn't know it was the kind of thing they did. Or maybe I seemed to be coping with it all so well that they were at their wits' end and had to resort to extreme measures to get some kind of reaction out of me.

Weight is obviously a sensitive issue. I always pride myself on being straight with my friends, but if I had a friend who I thought was morbidly obese, I wouldn't tell them my views if they seemed as happy as I had been. I've got really big friends now, but I'd never advise them to lose weight. You can't tell people to go on a diet. It doesn't work. Even though we should be able to speak to each other openly about this kind of thing, if you tell someone they're morbidly obese, you'll drive them straight to the fridge and they'll comfort eat.

You have to get a scare like I did or come to it of your own accord some other way. I'll always be a big girl, though. That's who I am. I don't have a problem with overweight people. I don't have a problem with myself – I have a problem with being 22 stone. I thought only house-bound Americans weighed 22 stone – not me, not Michelle. I was beautiful; I was sexy; I was the winner of *Pop Idol*. I didn't weigh 22 stone.

But I did.

Friday, 3 December 2004

Never again.

I was filmed having a colonic irrigation today. Gillian said she wouldn't let me start the programme until I'd had a complete clean out, because she wanted all the good food she's going to be putting in my body to be doing its job, instead of being clogged up with all the crap that's already there.

How in God's name can people enjoy this experience? The setting for this horrific crime was a beautiful clean room, with calming panpipe music and a truly lovely wee American woman, Margie, who, to look at, you would never have guessed could perform such an act. She said, 'OK honey, can you strip to the

---

COLONIC IRRIGATION

Colonics. Hah! Very odd things. While there is some debate about their health benefits – or whether they can even sometimes cause more harm than good – the basic principle is simple. The tube sends warm, sterile water into the colon (a bizarre feeling!) with the aim of flushing out excess mucus, gas, undigested food that's 'stuck' in there and whatever else happens to be hanging around. This is supposed to help the colon do its work better. The colon has two functions: it finishes off the digestive process, stores and then gets rid of the waste product, but it also absorbs whatever water, minerals and vitamins haven't already been taken in. Therefore, a 'clean' colon will do this last job better. Also, I was told that it can encourage weight loss (perhaps psychologically), give you more energy, and make your skin glow.

Possible risks of the procedure include tearing the colon, and the flushing out of the good bacteria that are there – often certain foods and supplements are recommended following a colonic to replace these.

Needless to say, neither the good nor the bad points are in the front of your mind when the lady is standing by with the tube!

waist?' I asked her if she meant up to the waist or down to the waist, and she said, 'You can leave your top half on.'

So I got up on the table and lay down. This time I'd insisted on a female camera operator because I couldn't have coped with Toby filming me having a colonic. OK, the guy had filmed me in a swimsuit, and I dealt with it really badly, but I'd coped with it. But I was not prepared for that guy to see me having a tube shoved up my bum; there was no two ways about it.

The camerawoman was so lovely, though – she was just like, 'Don't worry about it.'

First Margie had to do an internal examination – she put her fingers up my bum to make sure I'd not got any piles or anything.

And then I turned round to see her lubing up what looked like a slimline metal dildo. And I was looking at it, thinking, 'I'm not actually sure how comfortable I am with this.'

Throughout the whole experience, there was sweat pouring off me and I was thinking, 'I can't deal with this. I can't deal with this.' Thankfully the camera was on my face, so I just kept smiling through, but you'll be able to see the moment the tube went in – my eyebrows shot up and I made an 'oop' noise.

Margie said she was going to fill me up with water and when I felt I had to go to the bathroom I was to let her know. I thought she meant I was going to run out to the bathroom. So she pumped me full of water – ten minutes of hot water followed by ten minutes of cold, and you could really tell the difference. That cold water inside you ain't pleasant – it's freezing.

The next minute I thought, 'Oh my God.' I had that horrible diarrhoea feeling, the point of no return.

'I can't hold this in much longer,' I said.

'On you go,' she said.

'Pardon me?' I said.

'On you go.'

I had visions of it coming out everywhere, but obviously I didn't know how colonics worked and it all went shooting down this tube. And she had a mirror to show me what was coming out. I was almost heaving on the bed. 'Please take the mirror away,' I begged. It was just a sea of poo coming out of this tube.

Then it stopped and bubbles started coming out. She said, 'You must pass wind a lot.' I replied I didn't think I did more than the average person, but for twenty minutes there was just a stream of gas coming out of me.

This went on over and over for an hour. Then she removed the tube, stuffed my arse full of tissues and said that I should go visit the little girl's room at a fast pace: 'Run, honey, run!'

She wasn't kidding. What I hadn't worked out was that I still had loads of water up there. I got up, ran for the toilet (which was a mile from the room), leaking the whole way, sat down and the Niagara Falls came out of me for twenty minutes.

And I did feel a wee bit weak afterwards – but physically so much better.

It sounds stupid, but what had just happened was a whole cleansing ritual for me – and not just in the obvious way. What came out was not just shit, but the old me.

I came home and told Laura about it and she killed herself laughing.

Saturday, 4 December 2004

Day 1 of healthy eating, *You Are What You Eat* style.

Today was absolutely fantastic. I feel great and although celery is still absolutely disgusting I must persist with it. Went

Christmas shopping with Laura. She's also doing the detox with me. Life is wonderful.

Now my colonic has more or less cleaned me out, Gillian has put me on the *You Are What You Eat* eight-week detox, so that anything that goes into my body will do its job and then be passed out rather than clogging me up. The two-month detox is a process of flushing me out, basically. This will involve eating very pure foods – I'm not even allowed peppers or chillis because they're too spicy and can irritate the gut lining. During this time she wants my body to start functioning like a well-oiled machine, and to cleanse and change my palate and get me to accept health food.

THE EIGHT-WEEK *YOU ARE WHAT YOU EAT* DETOX

Detoxing is about clearing the body of the natural waste products that result following the consumption of substances such as caffeine, alcohol, tobacco, artificial food chemicals and refined sugars. Chronic illnesses and niggly health issues (such as poor digestion, tiredness, lethargy, dull skin and so on) are caused by a combination of nutritional deficiencies and from an over-loaded, 'over-toxified' body. The idea behind the detox is to 'purge' the body of these bad substances for a controlled period and give it what it needs instead – water to help eliminate the toxins, and nothing but the most nutritious fruits, veg and grains to provide the kidney, liver and bowels with what they need to do their job efficiently. Eating an abundance of fresh, wholesome, natural foods is the best way of doing this – so nothing artificial, no refined sugars and sweets, no junk food, alcohol, coffee or tobacco.

You should also aim to cut out dairy products during this eight-week period, particularly cow's milk, though it is worth consulting your doctor if you are worried about reducing your calcium intake. Ensure you keep up your calcium levels by eating plenty of broccoli, bony fish and nuts, all of which are good alternative sources. Cow's milk is difficult to digest for many people and can trigger allergic reactions such as eczema and asthma in susceptible individuals. It's also believed to make runny noses and mucus problems worse. Cows subjected to intensive farming methods are also exposed to antibiotics and other drugs that find their way into milk, so if you must eat or drink cow's products, always opt for organic. Good alternatives to cow's milk are sheep's or goat's milk, soya or rice milk.

As for what you *can* eat, there's plenty of it: all fruits, vegetables, fresh juices, wholegrains, pulses, herbs and seeds. You can also eat unprocessed proteins like lean white meat (e.g. simply grilled chicken or turkey with the skin removed), and fresh fish – especially oily fish, which is a great source of omega-3 fatty acids. Try to opt for organic or wild fish, as some farmed fish contain dyes and growth hormones. Avoid red meat and processed meat or fish during this eight-week period.

It's not necessary to go hungry on this detox, though you might find you feel worse for a while before you feel better, which is a sign that the body is beginning its recovery.

Remember, you might also crave junk food at first, but within a week or two your palate should have been retrained, so you'll find the detox easier to stick to as time goes by.

After the eight-week period is up, you can gradually start to reintroduce other foods.

Other things you can do to aid detox include:

- Always take your time over eating and chew thoroughly before swallowing. Don't eat on the hoof and listen to your body so you stop eating when you are no longer hungry.

- Try dry-skin brushing every morning – using a specialized brush with bristles made from natural vegetable fibres – always in the direction of your heart. This is believed to stimulate the lymph system, one of the body's main detoxification systems.

- Introduce more oxygen through your body by taking the time to do some deep, controlled breathing every day. This can assist the body's cleansing processes.

- Take regular exercise. Apart from all the well-known benefits, this can aid detoxing by keeping the bowel regular. Slow bowel movements mean that your poo remains in your body for a longer period, which increases the likelihood of any toxins in the poo being reabsorbed into your bloodstream.

Gillian has sent me detox menus for two weeks, which I'll combine in different ways for two months. Here is a typical detox day:

DETOX — TYPICAL MENU

First thing in the morning
1 cup of warm water + lemon
1 cup of peppermint tea

✯

Breakfast
Large bowl of blueberries

✯

Mid-morning snack
Celery, Cucumber and Carrot Juice

Push 2 celery sticks (washed and trimmed), 1 cucumber (washed and cut into thick strips) and 2 carrots (washed, topped and tailed) through a juicer.

✯

Go for a twenty-minute walk before lunch

✯

Lunch
Tuna and Rocket Salad

Drain 1 x 200g can of tuna in spring water and flake onto a bed of rocket (washed). Top with cherry tomatoes and a good handful of freshly chopped basil. Season with a squeeze of fresh lemon or orange juice and 1 teaspoon of extra virgin olive oil.

Mid-afternoon snack

Carrot and Apple Juice

Push 4 carrots (washed, topped and tailed) and 1 apple
(washed, cored and sliced) through a juicer.

✮

Dinner

Miso Soup with Spring Onions

Sprinkle a sachet of instant miso soup with tofu pieces into a
large mug. Add 1 spring onion, trimmed and finely chopped.
Top with hot water, stirring. (Save a tablespoon of the miso soup
to pour over the white meat for the main course.)

Chicken with Vegetables

Place an organic boneless chicken breast (skin removed), or
strips of organic turkey breast, on a piece of lightly oiled kitchen
foil and wrap loosely. Place on a baking tray and put in a
preheated oven at 200°C, gas mark 6, for 20 to 25 minutes until
cooked. Pour the reserved miso soup over the meat to moisten,
and serve with steamed carrots and broccoli, a big handful of
mung bean sprouts and a scattering of parsley or basil.

✮

Evening snack

1 or 2 fresh plums

This is a bit like cold turkey at times. When I look at people in the street they keep turning into walking bags of Doritos in front of my eyes. It's quite tough. Apparently, MSGs, E numbers and other flavour enhancers 'spoil' your palate, so when you go on a healthy-eating regime you can end up craving highly flavoured food. I'm told the cravings will subside after a while.

I'm really missing my fizzy drinks too, though I've learned that cola and diet cola also have an amazing amount of crap in them. Ordinary cola is basically carbonated water, sugar, caffeine and other flavourings – all rubbish, from a nutritional perspective. Even the carbonation of the water is bad, as it needlessly introduces dangerous carbon dioxide into the system. Diet cola isn't the answer either: it just swaps the sugar for artificial sweeteners to reduce the calories, though it still provides the sweet taste, which stops you 'retraining' your sweet tooth. It's also believed that artificial sweeteners can toxify your body and potentially cause allergy-like reactions and other illnesses in the long term.

A couple of years ago I was in Ibiza and there was a fisherman down there cleaning his boat with Coke, because it took the rust off. I'm not talking about a tiny bit of rust here, I'm talking about a great, thick layer of it, maybe two or three inches thick. I remember thinking, 'Jesus Christ, people drink litres of this stuff and it's ripping rust off a boat.' This was back before I was ready to change my life, though, so my solution was to switch to Diet Coke!

Sunday, 12 December 2004

The first week's gone really well and I haven't cracked once. The detox is hard going and sometimes I feel sick, which I'm told is a sign that the toxins are starting to leave my body, but I know it'll all be worth it in the end. And the best news is that I've lost 11 pounds in the first week of detox alone! That's almost a stone in a week. That's never happened to me before.

Gillian came over to deliver my Christmas hamper – and abuse me for four hours. She told me, 'You're going home for Christmas; it's going to be difficult; you cannot drink. Most people can have a couple of glasses of wine, but not you, not now. It's far too soon.'

I'm fine with it. I'm really going to do this now. The problem is that only one of my sisters knows about it, and my housemate, Laura – and that's it. What concerns me is not how I'm going to stop myself drinking over Christmas, but how I can get away with it without my family finding out. They'll think I've completely lost the plot.

Monday, 20 December 2004

I've arrived back in Glasgow and my family think I've been abducted by aliens because I don't want pizza on arrival. I still haven't told them about this because I want to do it on my own.

My cover story is that I've just decided to lose a bit of weight. I keep saying, 'Look, I just want to be a bit healthy just now.' And they've all seen that I've put on a lot of weight since *Pop Idol*.

I went out and bought the entire contents of my local fruit and veg shop, and a blender/juicer. *You Are What You Eat* is big on juicing, as it's a great way of getting fresh vitamins and minerals. Apparently it releases many of the nutrients that are bound in the fruit or vegetable's fibre, making it easier for the body to absorb. It's good for detoxing, because many of these nutrients are what the body has been lacking if it has been subjected to a typical junk-food diet. All juices are high in vitamin C and one glass of juice will count as one portion out of your five-a-day fruit and veg requirement. I've also found they taste surprisingly yummy!

SOME GOOD JUICES TO TRY

Apple
Protects the lungs against toxins, contains quercetin (which has shown anti-cancer properties)

Carrot
Rich in betacarotene, reputedly good for night vision

Celery
Reputedly a good liver tonic

Cranberry
Fights bladder infections, high in antioxidants

Grapefruit
Prevents eye cataracts, promotes weight loss by lowering insulin levels in the body

Orange
Useful quantities of calcium, vitamin C and folic acid

Pineapple
Anti-inflammatory, good for the skin, good for digestion

Pomegranate
Rich in iron, helps lower cholesterol; useful source of other minerals and antioxidants

Red grapes
Protects against heart disease, reduces blood pressure; a good detoxifier

I'm really charged up and ready for this. In fact, I made my favourite beetroot juice tonight, which is particularly good for boosting energy levels and the immune system.

Beetroot Detox Juice

Beetroot is rich in vitamins A, C and E and is regarded as a blood-improver, helping it to absorb essential nutrients and therefore boosting vitality and mental energy.

2 ready-prepared beetroots in their own juice, chopped roughly
4 carrots, washed, topped and tailed
4 sticks of celery, washed and trimmed
1 fennel bulb, washed and sliced

Put all the ingredients through a juicer. Pour and serve.

Thursday, 23 December 2004

I went out for the night with my friends and it was fantastic. All the guys that I used to work with at Scottish Power and the Marriott Hotel were there. And there was me on water all night. It felt weird, but also really good. A lot of people thought I was pregnant because I'd put on weight as well, and I was like, 'Chance would be a fine thing. I have no boyfriend! I just need to detox, guys.'

Saturday, 25 December 2004

Christmas Day!

I can't believe how easy this has been for me. I still don't know why I've stuck to it, but I didn't have a single drink. After the first two weeks of gagging, I'm really into my food now and enjoying being in control.

I filmed everyone for my *You Are What You Eat* video diary, but got away with it by saying I had a new video camera I wanted to try out.

Thursday, 30 December 2004

I'm off back to London today even though I've got to go up to Scotland again on 3 January. Mad I know, but I'd never get through Hogmanay without a whisky.

Saturday, 1 January 2005

19 stone 12 pounds

I've lost two stone. Two stone in a month. Unbelievable.

Happy New Year!

Everything's going great, although New Year's Eve was crap. All my mates were down from Glasgow, but thankfully they'd had a huge night the night before, so I didn't feel too bad about not drinking as no one else was really going for it either. I'd made some non-alcoholic mulled wine that Gillian had given me the recipe for, and then we went to this pub in St John's Hill. We were at home by 1 or 2 a.m. because it was rotten.

I don't think I'm more inhibited when I'm sober, but I just don't look as approachable. When I'm drunk it's whoooooo-hoooooo! Whereas you can see the hurt and distress on my face when I'm at a pub and not drinking. I just say, 'Water, please' in a choked-up voice.

Monday, 3 January 2005

I flew out to Glasgow this morning from London. My parents still know nothing about the show. I didn't eat on the plane and the stewardess looked at me as though I were wired to the moon.

My period is nine days late. It can't be that I've signed up for this show and I'm pregnant, can it? My period's never late. And that lovely bloke I met in Clapham was at the beginning of December . . .

Tuesday, 4 January 2005

It's my little sister's birthday today and Mum is having a family party. I need to go fully prepared, as she will have the usual pizzas, sausage rolls, potato salad, cheese, coleslaw and all the party food out on display. I'll take nuts, veggie juice, soup and haricot bean salad with my delicious basil and garlic dressing.

I spoke to Gillian about the fact that my period is now ten days late. Apparently, if you change your diet or lifestyle this can affect menstruation. So I can stop panicking about being up the duff.

Here is a recipe for a lovely dressing, which can help to liven up a green salad.

Basil and Garlic Dressing

(serves 2–3)

4 tsp of extra virgin olive oil
1 small garlic clove, peeled and crushed
1 tsp of fresh basil, finely chopped
1 tsp of cider vinegar (optional)

Lightly whisk all the ingredients together with a fork in a small bowl. Serve mixed with a handful of cooked beans or drizzled over freshly prepared salad leaves. Add a small amount of cider vinegar to taste.

Wednesday, 5 January 2005

I organized a lovely dinner party with friends in my Glasgow flat tonight and cooked for everyone. My dad is a god – he brought over loads of chairs for us. I made onion soup and then grilled salmon with steamed veg and potatoes, with apple pie to finish. Of course, I didn't touch the apple pie.

I finally saw the first signs of my period today.

Thursday, 6 January 2005

I looked back on my diary of four months ago today. I know I'm doing well, but I was obviously still completely drunk from the night before when I was thinking I'd be in a bikini eight months later . . .

Thursday, 13 January 2005

I'm back in London – got up this morning and felt great. I even managed to go on a two-hour walk.

However, I had an awful night at the pub with Sam Nixon this evening. It's the only time I've ever had a negative experience like it. We were minding our own business when a large, loud group of geeky lads sitting behind us – who thought they were cool, but weren't – started playing a game. You had to start at the beginning of the alphabet and say a celeb's name whose first and second name begins with the same letters, like Gareth Gates or Gina Gee or Sly Stallone. The person who messed up had to down their pint. When they got to M someone said, 'Martine McCutcheon', but another interrupted with 'Michelle McManus', and they all started laughing. Then this one cocky guy went, 'What? What? That can't count.' And the other guy said, 'She's a celebrity.' And cocky guy went, 'Well whatever, one-hit wonder. Where are you now, Fatty?'

Wee Sam, who's the height of shite, said, 'Right, that's it. I'm going to go and batter them.' And I said, 'Sit down.' I felt the tears welling up in my eyes. They must have known I was sitting behind them, but simply didn't give a toss. And if they didn't know at first, they knew by the time I got up to leave, about fifteen minutes later, because I looked at every one of them and they all looked back. But no one apologized or said anything. Some of them just sniggered a bit.

Sam got really upset but I just wanted to get out of there before I came off the still water and hit the wine to drown my sorrows. The old me would have got up and lamped that guy, saying, 'And here's a fat fist for you as well.' But what's the point? I went home and cried myself to sleep.

Why are people so horrible? I never did anything to hurt him.

I will prove him wrong.

Friday, 14 January 2005

19 stone 5 pounds

I've done it. I've lost well over 2 stone in six weeks – 2 stone 7 pounds.

I'm so glad I didn't wait till after Christmas to start this plan. I feel great – loads of energy and I'm so excited about losing all that weight already. I'm on a complete high and feel totally in control.

Sheryl – whose bridesmaid I was when I lost the weight during *Pop Idol* – arrives in London tonight for the weekend. She'll expect a big, boozy night. I'm not sure what I'll tell her about why I'm not drinking.

Saturday, 15 January 2005

Well, I had a lovely evening yesterday and drank six bottles of . . . *water*! Feel great. I'm loving not having hangovers.

Today's going to be a lazy day, as I've got a big night tonight with Sam Nixon and Chris Hide from *Pop Idol*. I think I'll curl my hair. Nights out are still big nights for me even though I'm not drinking, because instead of being out four evenings a week I'm staying in the whole time or going out walking. I don't trust myself to go out regularly and not be tempted to drink.

At first I was petrified of giving up alcohol. But I told myself that women get pregnant and give up for nine months all the time. I also remind myself that it isn't for ever, and the quicker I get this done the quicker I can get back on the booze again. That's the way I look at it. I do still think not drinking takes the fun out of life a bit, though. I can go out with my mates and have a great night, but I don't have as good a time as they do.

That said, I do still pull the same amount. It's just that the guys whom I pull when I'm sober are guys who approach me; the guys whom I pull when I'm drunk are guys *I* approach.

Sunday, 16 January 2005

I had a brilliant night last night, and although I wasn't drinking I had more energy than all my friends put together. I'm off to the cinema tonight to see *The Aviator* and we're walking, which should take about thirty or forty minutes. It's Baltic cold and my mate June's reminding me that she had to drag me down that hill on the twenty-five-minute walk at Ballycastle that I was so proud of back in September.

We went to lunch at the pizza chain Ask, which was a bit of a nightmare because there was nothing for me on the menu. I know you can order off-menu, so eating out shouldn't be a problem if you're on the *You Are What You Eat* plan, but I wasn't in the mood to make a fuss. I can't even eat goat's cheese or feta cheese at this stage because they're not pure enough for this detox part of the plan. Feta is very salty, apparently, and has only half the calcium of cheddar cheese. I ended up with a green salad, which was a bit boring, but I like eating out now and again – it makes me feel normal.

Monday, 17 January 2005

I got up quite early today as I had to take Sheryl to Liverpool Street. I opted for the train and tube, which also includes a twenty-minute walk back from the station. I can't believe how much I enjoy walking and using public transport these days.

Before I started this *You Are What You Eat* plan, I'd lived in London for a year and didn't know my way round at all – I just used to hop in cabs everywhere without thinking. Now I know every single tube line; I know exactly which one to use to get me somewhere. And walking as well – I know how to get from Oxford Street to Leicester Square to Covent Garden. It's all connected! Before, if I was in Covent Garden I'd have got a taxi to Leicester Square because I didn't know where it was, even though it's only a five-minute walk away.

Early to bed tonight, as I'm filming with Gillian in the morning.

Tuesday, 18 January 2005

The priority of the day is to please Gillian. Total surrender.

Filming with her went well. She was lovely and really pleased with my progress. Of course, no one knew beforehand whether I'd be able to lose any weight at all. She thinks I'm ready to join a gym, and Charlotte (my PA, assigned to me by 19 Management) and I will start visiting some soon.

And I got a present of skipping ropes from Gillian today. How lovely.

Wednesday, 19 January 2005

Another wonderful day. Charlotte came around and we filmed opening another of Gillian's presents. It was a trampette – a mini-trampoline. Charlotte tried it out and broke it on camera. It was a dodgy one anyway, but thank God it wasn't me who knackered it.

Saturday, 22 January 2005: Bristol

My friend June drove us to Bristol at 5 p.m. yesterday for my mate Vikki's thirtieth birthday party. I saw all my friends who were from Glasgow originally. I was very organized – I took my own dinner of brown rice with roast vegetables and drank water while everyone else sat round and downed glasses of white wine.

It's Vikki's actual birthday today, so about twenty-five of us went down to Bath for the day. I took a sachet of miso soup with me and asked the waiter for a bowl of hot water to dissolve it in and a side salad to go with it. Everyone else had pub grub – macaroni cheese, steaks and chicken – and of course in September I would have joined them, but now I'm so focused and I've lost two-and-a-half stone, so I'm sticking with healthy eating.

From the start I've always told people that they should eat what they like in front of me, though, because I have to get used to it.

Sunday, 23 January 2005

Today I went for a lovely walk around the countryside near Vikki's house. I even had to climb a hill – tricky, very tricky.

Although I'm fitter, hills still come as a shock because I didn't do any exercise at all when I was at my biggest. People always ask whether I felt short of breath, and the answer is I didn't because I never risked doing anything that might have had that effect on me. I was so lazy, I never found out. I had absolutely no energy before. Especially after a night out, I'd find it really difficult to get out of my bed. I'm one of these people who don't hear a thing once they're asleep. There could be a fire in the house, car alarms going off, someone getting murdered in the next room, and I would sleep soundly through the whole thing. I couldn't wake up in the morning either.

But now I wake up every morning at 7.30–8 o'clock because I've got so much more energy. I noticed that just as soon as I started healthy eating.

I'm still being very strict with my plan and I'm very proud of myself.

Monday, 24 January 2005

It snowed today.

I went swimming in the pool at the gym. It was so nerve-racking that I didn't make it anywhere near the gym itself. I can't even deal with thinking about that at the moment. I thought I'd be better at swimming, but I'd forgotten that you have to get almost naked to get into a pool, and once I was in there I was hopelessly slow, too slow even for the slow lane. I did twelve lengths of front crawl but still felt a little intimidated as most of the people there were fit. My stroke was lazy and there was a granny swimming with me in the slow lane who kept overtaking me.

All the women walk around naked in the changing rooms and most of them are in pretty good shape. I could never do that. I felt people were looking at me as though I didn't belong there – which is probably all in my head. I still felt uncomfortable, though.

Tuesday, 25 January 2005

Another great day. Went to aqua-aerobics with Charlotte. She's been brilliant. She's really assigned herself to me and does aqua with me and goes for walks with me in the middle of her working day. I'm thoroughly enjoying the aqua classes, actually. You don't feel like you're sweating when you're in the pool and you're supported by the water in all the moves you make, so it's harder to injure yourself. There were about ten of us in the class and we were made to do all sorts of stretches and jumps, which were made more difficult by the resistance of the water. You don't realize how hard you've worked till you get out of the pool. It's a great way for beginners to be introduced to the fitness world, as it's not as much of a shock to the system compared to other forms of exercise.

Afterwards, I went to 19 to pick up my single gold disc. I'm in a brilliant mood, what with that and the fact that the *You Are What You Eat* detox is going so well. I can't believe my eight weeks are nearly up. Once the detox part is over I'll be in the next phase of the plan, where I'm allowed gradually to introduce many of the banned foods and broaden the range of things I can eat – yippee!

I think I'll try to make tomato soup tonight.

Tomato and Basil Soup

Tomatoes are a 'superfood' because they contain an antioxidant called lycopene (which is found only in tomatoes and, in smaller amounts, in watermelon, guava and red grapefruit). Lycopene is one of the most powerful cancer-busting antioxidants around, and cooking tomatoes makes more of the lycopene available. They're also a good source of vitamins A and C.

8 large tomatoes, roughly chopped
1 tbsp of bouillon powder, or 1 organic vegetable stock cube
1 large clove of garlic, peeled and crushed
1 handful of fresh basil, roughly chopped
Freshly ground black pepper

Place the tomatoes, bouillon powder or stock cube and garlic in a medium-sized pan with just enough water to cover. Bring to the boil, then reduce heat to a simmer for 5 minutes. Take off the heat then pour the soup into a blender and process for a minute or so until it reaches a smooth consistency. Pour into a bowl, scatter over the chopped basil, season to taste with pepper and serve.

Friday, 28 January 2005

Today I'm filming for *You Are What You Eat* again, first with my new personal trainer Dax Moy and then at Borough Market.

I was introduced to Dax via Celador, the company that makes the show. He's such a lovely guy, in his thirties and good-looking, though he's very much the family man, which was one of the things I liked about him most. He kept showing me pictures of his family. I was so petrified of what he'd think about working with me that it didn't occur to me to fancy him.

Another thing that struck me about him was that he kept asking me what I wanted to get out of this, which no one ever had before. And he explained his reasons for getting me to do everything. When he introduced me to the cross-trainer (a type of machine, not a person!), he told me exactly which muscles it worked and what this would do for me.

He also looked at my body alignment by watching the way I moved and getting me to lift weights in the air. He concluded that the problem was I had a lazy arse. I could have told him that.

Then he got me to do some exercises to target my lazy arse, which seemed quite gentle at the time, but were agony in the morning. He'd warned me they would be.

He was sympathetic to my situation and I felt that I could work with him for a long time in the future. It was suggested that I see him two or three times a week, which I agreed to do. Some of his exercises are at the back of this diary.

Borough Market was fabulous and I got loads of beautiful fresh foods, like ginger, that I'd never added to my food before. Gillian told me that ginger assists digestion, and relieves flatulence, bloating and nausea, and in some African cultures it's considered to be an aphrodisiac. Very handy – if I had a boyfriend. But I didn't like the game – the rabbits and hares with their feet chopped off and skin and stuff. I couldn't be dealing with that. And the fish! With their eyes and teeth intact . . . ugh.

Anyway, I bought some lovely food – only to get home and find my fridge was broken. I rang the landlord and asked him to get a replacement fridge round here. He said he wouldn't even buy a thirty-quid fridge for me. 'I remember back in my day, we didn't even use fridges,' he told me.

'But back in your day you didn't charge a small fortune for an apartment, so get a bloody fridge round here quicksmart,' I replied. 'Don't be so ludicrous!'

He's mad and living in the Victorian age. When I first moved in he said he'd show me how to work everything. I thought he meant how to work the dishwasher, but instead he showed me how to put a plug into a socket.

Sunday, 30 January 2005

I walked with Laura to Lavender Hill and went health-food shopping – for things like hemp seed and bouillon powder, which you can get in Holland & Barrett or Fresh & Wild, but not all supermarkets. I'm learning so much about new foods. Hemp seed is apparently now seen as another 'superfood', as it contains lots of essential amino acids and omega-3 fatty acids. And bouillon powder is an organic alternative to veggie stock cubes, containing sea salt, which is slightly less unhealthy than normal salt, apparently. I can't believe how much I like that kind of stuff now I've been eating it for a couple of months. *You Are What You Eat* say that you should try to broaden the variety of foods you eat and not get stuck in a rut or be afraid to try new things. It's better for you from a nutritional point of view if you eat lots of different foods. It's true, I eat a far more adventurous diet now than before I started this plan.

I came home and made a huge salad. One of the benefits of the

You Are What You Eat regime is that you can eat as much of the foods they recommend as you like – unlimited supplies. Then I made some vegetable soup. Oh yes, I lead a very exciting life.

Below is a great nut salad – much tastier than it sounds! It combines all the goodness of nuts with that of the green stuff, and is brill if you're getting bored of the usual bog-standard salad.

Delicious Nut Salad

All nuts are excellent sources of iron, zinc and magnesium. They are high in protein as well as fat, although this fat is mostly monounsaturated or polyunsaturated (which can help lower blood cholesterol levels). Sesame seeds are also rich in beneficial minerals such as copper and calcium.

1 large bag of mixed salad leaves
1 bag of rocket leaves
10 cherry tomatoes, halved
1 large red onion, peeled and chopped
Half a red pepper and half a yellow pepper, washed and
    sliced, seeds removed
1 handful of raw cashew nuts (unsalted)
1 handful of raw hazelnuts (unsalted)
1 handful of sesame seeds

Place all the ingredients into a large salad bowl and mix well. Add a dressing of your choice; however, I would recommend 1 tablespoon of extra virgin olive oil with 1 teaspoon of chilli oil, or cider vinegar. (If you're on the first eight-week detox part of the *You Are What You Eat* plan, omit the chilli oil.)

Tuesday, 1 February 2005

I've been getting into this swimming lark – I did twenty-four lengths yesterday before having to get back home for the fridge repair guy.

Met a very nice man on a motorbike outside the aqua class afterwards. He was asking when my next single was out and saying that everyone missed me.

I spoke to Gillian as well, who said she'd send me some new menus because the first eight weeks of my detox are over!

I've got my first proper sessions with the personal trainer tomorrow. I'm nervous, but heigh-ho – it's got to be done. And in any case, I've got another mini-break in Spain to look forward to. We're going again in three days. Can't wait.

Wednesday, 2 February 2005

Gillian called me last night to talk about the next eight weeks. Now I'm allowed a heavier but still healthy lunch, perhaps with grilled chicken or fish – protein-based foods that I'll burn off at the gym – and a really light supper, like soup and a salad. I'm also allowed goat's cheese and feta cheese now!

The bad news, though, is I've been told to stay off the alcohol for the time being. Usually, you're allowed the odd glass of booze when you're off the eight-week detox and on the normal *You Are What You Eat* diet-for-life, but in my case Gillian reckons I'll fall off the wagon if I have so much as one drop of wine, so I have to keep avoiding it altogether. I've got so much weight to lose that the rules are a bit stricter for me.

NORMAL HEALTHY WEIGHT-LOSS DIET

Once the initial eight-week detox period is over, you can start to reintroduce some of the 'banned' foods gradually, though it's important to try to keep to the principles of healthy eating if you want to continue to feel the benefits – and especially if you are aiming to lose weight. You need to ensure your diet contains all the major groups of nutrients – carbohydrates, fats, proteins, minerals, vitamins, as well as fibre and water – and in the right proportions and quantities. Fruit and vegetables should form about a third of your diet and starchy carbohydrates (wholegrains and potatoes) should form another third. You can now gradually start to increase the amount of dairy (cheese, yoghurts and milk) in your diet, and reintroduce red meat occasionally.

Use your common sense: if you are trying to lose weight, you will need to be stricter about the amount of 'bad' foods you are reintroducing to your diet. However, if you're at your target weight and are more interested in a maintenance programme, opt for what Gillian calls the '80:20 rule' – in other words, eat the good foods 80 per cent of the time and allow yourself treats like the odd glass of wine or less healthy foods 20 per cent of the time.

Friday, 4 February 2005 to Monday, 7 February 2005: Spain

I had to get up at 3 a.m. on Friday to catch the flight out to Spain at 5.30 a.m., and felt like death. No one should ever get up at that time. Ever.

But as soon as I arrived in Salou it felt like I was home again. I love Spain.

It was difficult to eat much while I was out there because it's out-of-season and there are no restaurants open – only fast-food joints. I can't believe the contrast between this and the last time I came out here. Still, I've been doing lots of walking on the beach and instead of my usual boozy nights out we've been staying in and having fun with these brilliant Mexicana challenges. It's a females-only card game we all play. The stakes aren't the highest, but it's a great laugh. There's money to be won. There's nothing better than sitting round a table with a cracking good hand, thinking, 'You're going down.' You don't need booze to enjoy that feeling. I'm not promoting gambling, but I've included the rules here as it's a great diet distraction.

It's funny how different this holiday has been compared to previous ones. I'd usually have been drunk the whole time. Even my friends didn't drink as much this weekend because they felt too guilty for me. It made me realize I must have been the ringleader when it came to alcohol because they're not drinking nearly as much as they used to. Maybe it's because I'm not standing next to them with a gun to their heads shouting, 'DOWN THAT SAMBUCA!'

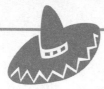

MEXICANA NIGHT

Mexicana (also known as Mexican poker) is a very enjoyable but highly competitive game of cards. You will need the following items to play:

- 2 packs of cards
- paper and pen
- money to gamble with
- extremely competitive players
- no alcohol

Background music is optional, however I would recommend the following:

- 'The Winner Takes It All' – ABBA
- 'Money, Money, Money' – ABBA
- 'I Want It All' – Queen
- 'The Gambler' – Kenny Rogers
- 'Money's Too Tight To Mention' – Simply Red
- 'Money For Nothing' – Dire Straits
- 'The Ace Of Spades' – Motörhead
- Anything Mexican or Spanish

Take the two packs of cards and shuffle them into one deck. Deal ten cards to each player (dealer should deal to the left), and put the remaining cards face down in one pile in the middle of the table. The dealer should then turn the top card face up and put it beside the pile in the middle. There are seven levels to Mexicana and the object of the game is to move through all seven levels, scoring the lowest number of points at the end of each round as possible. See below for levels and points system.

Level 1 2 sets of 3
Level 2 set of 3 and run of 4
Level 3 run of 7
Level 4 2 runs of 4
Level 5 set of 4 and run of 4
Level 6 3 sets of 3
Level 7 2 sets of 4

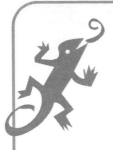

Points
Cards numbered 3–9 = 5 points
Cards numbered 10, J, Q and K = 10 points
Ace = 15 points

Wild Cards
Card numbered 2 = 20 points
Joker = 25 points

The person to the left of the dealer will start the game and must first pick a card from the middle of the table either from the pile or the card facing upwards if it helps their hand later. If they have the complete sets/runs required of the level they should put the hand down for the rest of the players to see, but they can still add to them. If you can't make the required hand from your cards, simply throw away a card you do not want in disgust (usually the card with the highest points) to the middle of the table face up and the game moves on to the next player. The sets and runs can be made of any suits as long as they are the same numbers, i.e. all 3s or two 3s and a Joker, although you must have all the sets or runs for the particular level before you can put your hand down on the table.

Note: you cannot throw away the two wild cards. It's also worth mentioning that you also shouldn't throw away cards that may help the player to your left, for example; if they are on level 2 and have a run of 4 consisting of 4, 5, 6, 7, you should not throw away an 8 or a 3. You should hold on to this as you will be able to 'blow' these cards on to other players' hands when your set/run is down.

The first person to get rid of all their cards ends the round and players must tally up the points for their remaining cards. If you managed to get your hand down then you move on to the next level. If not, you must remain on that level and everyone else moves on.

Drinking alcohol is not recommended as the more drunk you get, the worse you play, the more money you lose and the more violent you become.

Everyone chucks a pound (or ten) in at the beginning. Whoever wins all the rounds wins the money.

Tuesday, 8 February 2005: London again

Friends who stayed overnight after the flight yesterday evening all left at lunchtime, and I went straight to the gym. Did twenty laps in the pool.

I've just found out there will now be two *You Are What You Eat* shows – one in June and one in December. That's a great incentive for me and my healthy eating – June's only four months away.

I've started my Spanish lessons again.

Adios amigos.

Thursday, 10 February 2005

I flew to Glasgow today to see the mighty Green Day in concert. They were fantastic. Would have thrown my knickers onstage if I could have got them off in time. If Billy Joe Armstrong could hurry up and propose to me, that would be great.

Got some rather cheeky text messages from Gillian today saying stuff like, 'Why have you not got in contact with me? Have you fallen off the wagon?' Got really fed up as I am trying very hard to get through this and need her to get off my case.

Saturday, 12 February 2005

It's really hard to keep this eating plan under wraps because everyone's starting to notice now. People are beginning to say, 'Look, what the hell's going on?' It's normal not to drink in January, but not for this long.

I'm off to London today with my gran and my mum in tow. They can also see a big difference and it's getting harder to lie to them about the show. I'm not going for dinner with them tonight, so I can make my own food at home – it's easier that way.

Sunday, 13 February 2005

I was up bright and early this morning and went to Mass with Gran and Mum. I like to believe there's someone there, that when I die I'm going to go somewhere, and if I need help sometimes I can talk to somebody.

Later on, everyone else had a full cooked breakfast while I had grilled salmon with sage.

Then we decided to see the film of *The Phantom of the Opera*. I didn't want Gran, aged seventy, to have the hassle of the tube, so I booked a cab for Leicester Square at 7.40 p.m.

It didn't turn up.

So we got on a bus to Clapham Junction to get a taxi from there.

There were no cabs.

I looked at Mum and Gran and thought, 'The only way we can physically get to Leicester Square in twenty minutes is by train and tube.'

'Right, girls. We have to get our skates on,' I said.

So I ran ahead and bought all the tickets. We got on the train to Waterloo and then the tube to Leicester Square. I told them I was going to go on ahead to buy all the cinema tickets and asked them what they wanted to eat.

Gran: 'Ooooh, a hot dog? Ooooh, I don't know.'

Me: 'DOYOUWANTAHOTDOGORNOT?'

Then I ran from the tube station to Leicester Square, got all the tickets, the food and a bottle of water for myself.

When they arrived at the cinema, my mum and gran were just staring at me, my mum practically with tears in her eyes.

Me: 'What? What's wrong?'

Mum (slowly): 'What's happened to you? You ran. You sprinted. In twenty-four years, I've never seen you run.'

I was thinking, 'Holy shit. I ran. And I didn't even feel out of breath, I didn't feel tired. I didn't even think about it.'

And I sat in the cinema that night with a huge smile on my face, thinking, 'I ran.'

Monday, 14 February 2005

The day all singletons dread.

I got up and got out this morning, leaving Mum and Gran in bed. Later I came back and took the ladies out to lunch and then to the nail bar, where they had their feet done. And then we had a nice walk home.

The two of them left in the evening with Mum saying she couldn't believe the difference in me. She said that she'd never seen me walk anywhere, let alone run. Hurray!

No cards to or from me. And my flatmate Laura has just split up with her boyfriend, so we stayed in and watched the two *Bridget Jones* films. Laura did a bottle of wine. I rang my friend Carrie today and she had her voicemail on, saying, 'Don't contact me as I'm single and it's Valentine's Day. Speak to you tomorrow.'

Wednesday, 16 February 2005

I came home to celebrate with Laura, as she's got a new job as PA to the chief executive of her company. I booked my mum and dad a holiday today, too. Even though I'd looked forward to paying off their mortgage when I won *Pop Idol* and they only had a couple of grand to go on it, they wouldn't let me. They won't let me give them any cash either. The only thing I can do is book them a holiday, because that doesn't feel like money to them. I have to plan the whole thing for them and just hope they can get the time off work.

My sisters are a different story. They would quite happily rob me blind. When I'm in Glasgow I have to keep one eye open when I'm sleeping at night.

Thursday, 17 February 2005

I went to the gym for my first yoga class today, on Gillian's recommendation. It was tough, but I was determined to stick with it. I found the Downward Dog pose and the Salute to the Sun difficult . . . and, basically, everything else as well. To be honest, I didn't get as much out of it as seeing Dax or going to my aqua class because I don't have the flexibility of the people around me. Plus, I have the attention span of a two-year-old and find it impossible to shut my mouth for the length of a whole class.

There was an old woman there who was like an elastic band. She was unbelievable. I was so humiliated that, at the age of twenty-four, I have no flexibility whatsoever. In fact, I'm aching quite badly now, but I'll get over it.

Nicki told me that on 2 March, Channel 4 are going to announce my *You Are What You Eat* appearance in a press launch about their new programmes for the summer. I felt sick. There's only a couple of weeks to go and I haven't even told my family yet. I still don't feel ready to do that. They'll think my management has forced me into it because I've always been so happy with myself up till now. I don't want to make them worry about me.

Friday, 18 February 2005

I got up and went for Round 2 of yoga. Now I'm really in agony. But I'm going shopping to cheer myself up this afternoon and am meeting my friend Nic at 6 o'clock.

I went to the pub and drank water this evening. I felt so guilty for Nic, because she was looking for a really big girls' night out, but I couldn't explain what was happening. I couldn't lie though, either. In the end I broke and told her about the show. Strange, because she's one of the people I haven't seen for ages. She said, 'Wow!' and told me I looked amazing, and totally accepted that I wasn't drinking after that.

I've been thinking a lot recently about the press launch being released and the reaction I'm going to get. I'm really scared people are going to slag me off and say I've sold out. Maybe I have. I don't even know any more. During *Pop Idol* I was seen as a role model for larger women and I was proud of that, but since I weighed in at 22 stone I feel like I'm just promoting obesity. Being a big girl and being 22 stone are two different things. I don't want to advertise being morbidly obese and I feel like that's what I'm doing, even if I don't mean to.

Sunday, 20 February 2005

A girls' day out. Celtic are playing Rangers today, so the ladies are on a tour of various pubs in Clapham Junction watching the football. Started in O'Neill's, then the Slug and Lettuce, then the Happy Drinker, then the bowling alley in Kingston – long story. Normally I would have spent the whole day drinking pints, but instead I drank water and nettle tea (which I took out with me because I'm getting so sick of water). Oh, how the mighty have fallen.

What I've learned since December is that drunk people can be a real pain to deal with and what's more they talk shite. It's hilarious the way their eyes change when they've had a few. I've noticed that if you're with a group of drunk people – say, there are seven in your group – two of them don't have a clue what you're saying at any given point because it's taking their full concentration to keep their eyes open.

And drunk people will keep going all night – whereas if I get to 2 o'clock and I've not pulled, I know I'm not going to find any of them attractive without my beer goggles.

Gillian is still doing my head in with her text messages. I'm going to have to say something to her. She keeps going from one extreme to another – one minute she's sending messages saying how proud of me she is, and the next she's accusing me of falling off the wagon.

We ended up in the bowling alley because my friend Linda fancied one of the guys she worked with in Asda. She dragged us all to Kingston by telling us it was one stop on the tube. It isn't. It isn't anywhere near a tube station.

And I got mobbed, because all the wee kids were like: 'MIIICHEELLE MCMANNUUUUUS!'

I was thinking, 'I'm going to stab you, Linda.'

So, a big fan base in Kingston, apparently.

Monday, 21 February 2005

Gillian is coming to the house to film tomorrow, so I've got to clean, especially in my bedroom, as that's where they'll be filming.

Linda and I decided to do some DIY in my flat. Never again. The landlord tried to do some rewiring himself to save money and we had no electricity in the bathroom. We spent six hours with a flashlight trying to fix it. By the end it was working, but you had to be careful not to touch the wire.

Tuesday, 22 February 2005

Filming with Gillian starts.

I was up and dressed and ready at the crack of dawn, because Gillian was on her way. Emma, who's standing in as director for Ita today, and Kevin, who also works on the show, arrived at 9 a.m.; everyone else came at 10.

We had a great day filming and it started to snow while Gillian and I were rollerblading in the park. I'd never done rollerblading before and I hated it. I think Gillian wanted to show people that when it comes to fitness you don't have to pay an enormous gym membership, because you've got this wonderful facility around you, which is free – the great outdoors.

I reckon she also wanted to show off her rollerblading skills – although she was pretty unsteady too – and unfortunately

I'm too vain for rollerblading. Unless you look like Lara Croft, you just look like an idiot. I looked more like the Incredible Hulk in my green cold-weather gear, helmet and kneepads.

I met June, Lynsey and Nicola for dinner. Lebanese – love it. It's the kind of thing I would never have touched before, but I was introduced to it because of hummus and falafel and things like that, which are recommended on the *You Are What You Eat* plan. Still, I only eat Lebanese food very occasionally as it contains a lot of bread, crushed wheat and rice – I used to eat so many really heavy carb-based foods, and now my diet is so much lighter that when I eat lots of carbohydrates I end up feeling too full.

OTHER FOODS I'D NEVER HAVE THOUGHT I'D BE EATING A YEAR AGO

Quinoa (pronounced 'keen-wa') – a very strange substance. It looks like a rice or couscous dish but tastes of not much at all, just a bit nutty. It's low in carbs and high in protein, and a great substitute for rice, especially if you like curries but can't have chicken and rice together because of the 'don't mix carbs and protein' rule. Worth a shot! The grains are rich in iron and high-quality protein, and are a useful source of calcium and B vitamins. It's also gluten-free, so many people find it easier to digest than other grains that contain gluten, such as wheat, rye, spelt and barley.

Miso soup – my favourite soup of all time now! You can buy this in packet form or make your own (see Laura's miso soup recipe, page 199). It's found in Japanese restaurants but is incredibly easy to make – you just dissolve a sachet in boiling water and you can put in some extra chopped tofu and spring onion to liven it up. It's made from fermented soya bean paste and is eaten almost daily in Japan, where it's been touted for centuries as a remedy for weak digestion, cancers, low sex drive and more.

Seeds – no, not bird seeds, although they look the same! All seeds – sesame, linseed, pumpkin, sunflower, hemp and so on – are highly recommended on the *You Are What You Eat* healthy-eating regime and I'm a big fan, especially when they're added to a salad. Sprinkle a handful of seeds over your salad to give it that extra kick. It really does make a difference. All seeds and nuts are rich in omega-3 fatty acids and also some trace minerals that are often missing in our diet, such as zinc and selenium, which, among other things, are essential for a healthy immune system.

Beans – not baked! Haricot, flageolet, cannellini, mung, aduki, kidney – the list is endless and all are highly recommended on the plan. Again I found these beans quite tasty, although be warned: if you're adding them to a casserole or salad, read the packet first as most beans need to be soaked overnight in cold water. Preparation is essential. Beans are rich in dietary fibre, which bulks out your poo and promotes a healthy, cleansed bowel. They're also a superb source of protein if your diet is low in meat or fish (for example, if you're a veggie). They also help the heart, as they lower cholesterol, and they're rich in complex carbohydrates. Aduki beans are particularly good – Gillian calls them the 'weight-loss bean', and in Japan they're thought to have healing properties.

Seaweed – this is one of the richest natural sources of vital minerals. Seaweed is high in calcium, iron and other minerals such as iodine. The Japanese love their seaweed – and they're among the healthiest (and longest living) people in the world. Because seaweed is harvested from the sea, it's a natural product that hasn't been subjected to fertilizers or pesticides. There are lots of different types, with names like nori, wakame, kelp, arami and dulse. Among their many benefits, they promote weight loss, cleanse the blood and eliminate water retention. Another superfood.

Saturday, 26 February 2005

My family arrived from Glasgow yesterday morning. They still don't know I'm doing the show, so I've had to be careful.

They arrived safely at 11 o'clock and we went to Harrods for the afternoon, where they bought Krispy Kreme donuts and I had a smoothie. Felt surprisingly fine about it.

This morning I woke up and made everyone a fried breakfast – except myself, of course. It sounds harder than it is. I've discovered by accident that when I cook the fry-up, smelling it all the while, by the time I come to eat it, I feel full. I'm brilliant at cooking fry-ups, even if I say so myself, and if I put one down in front of them and they enjoy it – and I sound like my mum here – that's enough for me. I had a pint of my favourite mango, banana and orange smoothie instead.

In the evening, I went to watch *Ant and Dec's Takeaway* show being filmed live. I'm really good friends with Lisa, who's my make-up artist and Ant's fiancée. Obviously, I know the boys themselves from *Pop Idol* – and they are as lovely as you'd expect. We got our VIP passes, and me and the girls – my two wee cousins – went backstage. Those boys totally deserve to be where they are today because they are so unaffected by their fame and success.

Mango, Banana and Orange Smoothie

This is a delicious drink and full of goodness. Bananas are rich in potassium, which is good for your kidneys; mangoes are rich in many vitamins, and – unusually for fruits – are a good source of the mineral copper (which helps the development of healthy bones, heart and skin); and oranges have many benefits, the most well known being that they are full of vitamin C. If you can go for blood oranges, even better, as these contain anti-oxidants that may offer protective benefits against internal diseases such as intestinal cancers.

1 large mango, peeled, stoned and roughly chopped
2 bananas, peeled and roughly chopped
2 whole oranges, peeled and quartered

Place all the ingredients in a blender or food processor.
Blend together for a few seconds and serve. Simple!

Monday, 28 February 2005

18 stone 2 pounds

Aaaaaaaaaaargh! Why have I stopped losing weight? I've been the same weight for at least two weeks now. It's really annoying. I've followed the rules. I haven't been slacking from the plan. What should I do? Must speak to Gillian about it.

Filming with Gillian was cancelled today, so I went to the gym and then for lunch with Amelia, my mate from *Pop Idol*. She was a researcher on it. It was a real ego boost, as I haven't seen her since September, and she nearly died when she saw me. I love that reaction.

Tuesday, 1 March 2005 (Rabbits, rabbits, rabbits)

I'm going to my first Pilates class today, as recommended by Gillian. I was very excited about it beforehand, as Gillian reckons it will do me the world of good and give me a washboard tummy. The other day she pulled up her top and showed me her own amazing abs, which she got from Pilates. I found the class better than yoga, but it still wasn't really my thing – lots of lying around on mats and trying to engage muscles I don't even think I have. It didn't make me break into a sweat and I just felt self-conscious lying there. I don't think I'll go back.

I'm starting to get quite nervous about the press release tomorrow and telling my family. I think I'll ring my mum tonight.

Wednesday, 2 March 2005 (D-Day!)

Well, it's all out in the open and now I'm scared about what the reaction will be. My family were fantastic, as expected, but now I have to face the media. I keep telling myself I don't give a stuff, but in the same breath I hope they're not too nasty. I'm putting a statement out on the website today as I want the fans to hear it first.

I told Mum and it turns out she's been worried sick for three months. In November the results of my medical for the show had turned up – in Glasgow. Mum had rung and said, 'You've got medical results here. What are they for?' and I'd told her, 'You know I'm on the Pill and I just decided to get checked out.'

When I explained about the show, she revealed to me that she'd thought I'd got devastating news at the medical, which was why when I came home for Christmas I wouldn't eat or drink anything unhealthy. She'd thought I'd have to have some kind of terminal illness for me not to drink – that's what my family think of me!

Thursday, 3 March 2005

Not too much press this morning, so that was good. I'm happy they didn't pick up on it too much.

What upset me, though, was *The Wright Stuff*. I was in the gym when it came on. One of the actors from *Fat Friends* was a guest on the show and he slated me for doing *You Are What You Eat*, even though he's overweight himself. He of all people should know what it takes to make that kind of decision. He was just horrible, which is such a shame because I thought he was a decent enough actor.

He thought I was using my weight as a publicity stunt, but even if I was – which I'm not – what does it matter to him? And he makes a living out of his weight – he's in a show called *Fat Friends*!

Matthew Wright pretended not to know who I was, even though I was a guest on his show only a year ago.

Monday, 7 March 2005

I went to my friend June's house on Friday, as she was off work sick, and took her some goodies: miso soup that I'd made, salmon with pesto crust (see recipe on page 149), and a bottle of Lucozade (I'm sure Gillian would disapprove of the latter, but isn't it traditional if you're unwell?).

The miso soup must have worked. June had recovered by Saturday and we went to the Savoy Hotel in London on a manhunt. We drank non-alcoholic cocktails and met a lovely boy, whom I'll call H. He spent the evening with us and we swapped numbers. We've been texting ever since.

I weighed myself yesterday and I've finally lost some weight again: I'm 17 stone 11 pounds now.

I went for my first driving lesson – on a simulator – today. Very scary, but I thought that I'd turn the fact that I'm not drinking into a positive step and learn to do something new.

Tuesday, 15 March 2005

I arrived in Dublin on Saturday morning for a hen night in the evening – I love this place. Drank thirty small bottles of water.

I wonder whether Celador will be disappointed? Did they expect to see the old boozing Michelle again? They lent me a camera so I could film it!

On Sunday I met up with Brian Ormond (who is now presenting for Irish TV channel RTE) and my friend Trevor. They said I looked fab. I stayed on another day because Brian took me to see *Blood Brothers* at the Gaiety Theatre on Monday night. Gillian texted me to ask what fish I eat. Hello, G? You tell *me* what I eat!

In the old days, fish and all creatures from the sea were strictly off the menu. I couldn't stand the smell, the taste, the texture and most of all the look, especially if the fish was still intact – teeth, eyes and all. It was a psychological thing, of course. Once I'd overcome my fear, I was ready to try more and more types of fish. On the *You Are What You Eat* show, they called the tuna Gillian offered me a 'hateful plateful of Michelle's worst nightmare – fish'. I tried it and said, 'Actually, it's not that bad.' I love it now.

A couple of months down the line we had a bit of a row on camera. I was only eating two types of fish at the time, tuna and salmon, and Gillian thought I'd either get bored of them and give up on fish altogether, or just stick with those two fish and never try any others. But although I was only eating two types of fish, at least it was two more than I had been eating before. I thought she was being impatient. She said she thought I was in a rut again, and I couldn't believe she hadn't noticed all the changes I had made to my life and that I was trying really hard. She kept saying, 'It's not about the fish, Michelle.' She was right, I thought. It was about her not being positive enough, in my view.

Here are my current Top Ten fish:

1. Salmon
2. Tuna
3. Monkfish
4. Halibut
5. Sea bass
6. Dover sole
7. Turbot
8. Trout
9. Cod
10. Lobster (technically a crustacean, but I love it!)

FISH: THE FACTS

My new love of fish was great news for my healthy lifestyle. Eating fish – if possible, at least twice a week – reduces the risk of heart and cardiovascular disease, which is especially important if you're overweight. Fish is low in saturated fat, low in total fat, and is an excellent source of protein and vitamins D and B – in short, it's a nutrient-dense food. Some fish are particularly rich in omega-3 fatty acids, a highly beneficial fat thought to help lower cholesterol (and again, therefore, help the cardiovascular system). Other studies show that omega-3s help prevent arthritis and relieve depression.

All fish contain some omega-3, but in general the 'fattier' the fish, the more omega-3 there is. Good sources include salmon, mackerel, herring, tuna and anchovy. White fish, such as cod and haddock, contain lesser amounts of omega-3 but are still a good source of protein, vitamins and minerals, such as iodine.

White fish has one advantage over oily fish – it contains far fewer calories. I've found that if I eat fish three times a week, a good balance is to have a couple of portions of oily fish and one portion of white; loads of omega-3s, but you're still watching the calories.

I'm heading home now – shattered. H sent me a book he'd told me about at the Savoy, all beautifully gift-wrapped. How sweet.

Wednesday, 16 March 2005

Curses! How on earth have I put on 4 pounds? I'm hopping. It turns out that the scales are wonky and making up their own mind. I spent the rest of the afternoon beating the living daylights out of the scales.

I need new scales.

H texted again. Big date on Sunday.

Sunday, 20 March 2005

Whooo hooo! H texted me at 9.30 this morning – 'Just off to play golf, really looking forward to seeing you tonight. See you about 7.30 p.m.' He's keen. Good sign.

Out shopping on Oxford Street this afternoon and H texted me at 5 p.m. to cancel. He said that his sister was ill and could he postpone? I think he was too drunk to call so he texted. My theory is he went to the golf club all day and just got steaming. Men are very rubbish. I really liked this one. I've absolutely no idea what happened.

Tuesday, 22 March 2005

Oh my God, *Star* magazine have just made mine the 'worst bottom' of last year and my huge arse is on the front cover. Aaargh! I nearly fainted. They actually had the cheek to blow up my arse. I mean, it's big enough. There's no need. Bad *Star* magazine.

Wednesday, 23 March 2005

I went to meet Kate Thornton for lunch. She was looking so well. She's just flying high with her new job – on *The X Factor* – and her new man.

I came home and there was a paparazzo waiting for me; he caught me going for my driving lesson. They're starting to want pictures of me again because of the press release about *You Are What You Eat*, and because I've lost a bit of weight.

MICHELLE'S GUIDE TO MEDIA MANAGEMENT

Tricks journalists use:

1. Silence. After you've answered a question they stay quiet so that you panic and fill the gap with the first thing that comes into your head – usually some terrible crime you've committed or a damaging secret about another *Pop Idol* contestant. Beat them at their own game: silence them right back.
2. Laughing at things you say in an attempt to ingratiate themselves with you. Even when you know your joke wasn't that funny. Or when you've not made a joke at all, which is downright alarming.
3. Lying.

Friday, 25 March 2005

I flew up to Glasgow yesterday. Went to the dentist to have my terrible teeth fixed and then ate baked halibut with veg at the swanky hotel and restaurant, One Devonshire Gardens. My little sister's doing my hair for me today.

Five o'clock: colonic irrigation – scary thought. Actually, this time it wasn't too bad – although I missed the film crew, obviously. Linda, the lady with the tube, was really sweet and spent a lot of time explaining the benefits of the colonic and exactly what was going to happen – how could I forget? I could have done with some of this advance preparation last time, when it all came as a bit of a shock!

As a result, I was surprisingly relaxed about having a tube inserted in my backside on this occasion. And believe me, you don't want to be uptight for that experience. I feel like one of those LA women who has colonics all the time.

Lynsey had a party this evening, but I'm in bed at eleven o'clock. Basically, I just couldn't handle the sight of everyone drinking. I really wanted a drink tonight. I made myself a raw veg juice and drank it with a completely sour face, and then went to bed.

Everyone was like, 'She looks great, but she's a bitch.'

Saturday, 26 March 2005

Mum held a little get-together for the family and I made everyone salad with my cider vinegar and garlic oil dressing. They loved it.

Cider Vinegar and Olive Oil Dressing

1 tsp of cider vinegar

3 tsp of extra virgin olive oil

1 garlic clove, peeled and crushed

**Put all the ingredients in a bowl and mix together.
Drizzle over salad.**

I went out to watch Scotland play Italy in a World Cup qualifying match. I ended up in Carrie's flat with a smoothie at 9 p.m. on a Saturday night.

Rock on.

Sunday, 27 March 2005 (Easter Sunday)

My mum is the best. She bought me a massive basket of fruit instead of an Easter egg. It was all tied up with pink ribbons and everything. I love her. However, I drank 3 litres of water today and no doubt will be on the toilet all night. I'm very happy, though – the *Sunday Mail*, a paper in Scotland, did a lovely article on me and pointed out how much weight I've lost.

Thursday, 31 March 2005

I had to rearrange my Tuesday flight back from Glasgow today because of flu. Still bunged up now. I also had to cancel filming *You Are What You Eat* yesterday, and Gillian called to make sure I wasn't faking it. Honestly, I'm not well!

I decided I must step up a gear now – on the cross-trainer, particularly – because it's eight weeks until the show broadcasts, and my long-awaited holiday. I need to be in a bikini.

I had a driving lesson and went home and made soup, pesto and hummus.

Given my bad luck with men lately, my friends and I are compiling a psycho table.

PSYCHO TABLE

Every single woman should have one of these as a point of reference. Not only will it remind you of what you're dealing with when it comes to men, but it will also reassure you that it is never, ever your fault. Not even a little bit. (Names have been changed to protect the guilty.)

NAME	LENGTH OF TIME DATED	BREAK-UP METHOD	REASON	PSYCHO MARKS (OUT OF 10)
George	Two months	Email	Not ready for commitment – even though he said 'I love you' after two weeks (I never said it!)	7
H	Texted constantly for two weeks	Stopped texting	Arranged a date and said his sister was sick, so had to reschedule – never heard from him again	8
Dom	Three months – two dates and approximately 200 text messages	He got caught	Had a girlfriend, even though he'd texted two or three times a day for three months, telling me how much he fancied me	10
Jay	Six weeks	Over dinner	Going on holiday with his mates and wanted to take time to think about our relationship. (In other words, he wanted to shag around for a week.) Wanted to get back together after his holiday	9

Friday, 1 April 2005

Did an hour of exercises when I woke this morning. Then this evening I went out in central London with some people from Laura's work and drank water. I had quite an audience all night, because Laura had told them all that I was doing *You Are What You Eat*, so they all pinned me up against the wall: 'What's Gillian like?' 'What are you doing?' 'What do you have to eat?' One guy wanted me to write the detox rules on his arm.

Saturday, 2 April 2005

Today I went for a walk up to Clapham's Northcote Road with Laura, and spent sixty smackers on lilies (Elton John, eat your heart out). Flowers are the latest thing for me to spend my money on, now that I'm not drinking. My home looks like a funeral parlour (RIP the old Michelle who used to drink!).

I went to the Savoy Hotel on a manhunt again this evening. Things had started off so well with H that I just had to go back for more.

I'm really starting to get down about being constantly sober when all I want to do is purchase a box of white wine, lie underneath it and open the tap and my mouth.

I thought about having a drink at the Savoy because last time I had non-alcoholic cocktails and this time I thought maybe they could slip a bit of spirit in. I'm pleased to say that I resisted the temptation, though.

Monday, 4 April 2005

I'm never going shopping again. I was out from 10 a.m. till 7.30 p.m., but the good news is that I've got an outfit from

Planet for my friends Anne and Wayne's wedding, and everything is a size 18! Hurray! This is the first time in my adult life I've been that size. It feels amazing. And I have to say, I look great in the dress. It's white cotton with black and green flowers and black straps. I'm going to wear it with a green cardie, Fifties-style shoes and a bag to match.

Still, I've hit another plateau. I'm not losing weight at the moment.

Wednesday, 6 April 2005

The filming schedule for *You Are What You Eat* is picking up speed now. Yesterday involved shooting me shopping at the organic supermarket Fresh & Wild, then the fish shop in Wandsworth, south London, and then at New Look on Oxford Street. I'm shattered. Today we were filming again with Dax Moy, my personal trainer, and tonight the crew recorded a dinner party at my house. I cooked sea bass in a pesto crust with lots of veg (see recipe on page 149).

It was a good party, because none of my friends drank all night. Even when the film crew left – there was no drink in the house. There was no change in the conversation. They all commended me on my cooking, but after that we talked the same old crap, with Trevor going, 'Bejesus, I can't get a man.'

Saturday, 9 April 2005

I weighed myself yesterday morning and I'm 17 stone 6 pounds. Whooo-hooo! I was 21 stone 12 pounds when I started on the *You Are What You Eat* plan. It's amazing.

Today was the big day – my friends' wedding. The sun was shining and I have to say, I looked good – all tanned and a size 18. The best bit was that my boobs looked huge in this dress! However, I was literally the only single person at the wedding. Spent the whole day sitting and thinking, like Bridget Jones, 'Oh my God, I will die alone and be eaten by Alsatians.' It will happen to me. At least I look bloody great. I had a soup and some veg for the meal.

Sunday, 10 April 2005

I had a fab day yesterday, regardless of my single status. Everybody kept telling me how wonderful I looked, which was lovely.

It was a chilled day today before I headed back to London. Nic's mum Jackie cooked everyone Sunday roast and made me chicken with veg separately. She's so sweet. Sunday roast is a religion up north. I said I can't eat any of that, I'm sorry. So she went out and bought me two skinless chicken breasts, steamed some vegetables and poured over it some bouillon stock that I'd brought with me.

Wednesday, 13 April 2005

Today I read a really shitty letter in *Star* mag. This girl – Clare Smith from London – had written: 'Michelle's bum in last week's issue was a sad sight. Stop eating Chelle.' Why are people so awful? I would love to see Clare Smith from London's arse up close, then blown up to A4 size. Bitch. No one's arse in a swimsuit blown up to that size is going to look that good.

Friday, 15 April 2005

I have to stop weighing myself every day. It's getting depressing. I remind myself that *You Are What You Eat* is not about weighing and scales but a whole new lifestyle, which I've certainly got.

Mum and Maria went home after spending a few days with me in London, and Lynsey and I went to the gym. Lynsey was quite shocked at how fit I was.

I had a very lazy night, and Lynsey and I St. Tropezed. Because there's less of me, it's amazing how much longer a bottle lasts now I've lost weight.

OTHER WAYS OF GAUGING HOW MUCH WEIGHT YOU'VE LOST WITHOUT USING SCALES

1. Noticing how loose the seatbelt is on a plane.
2. Checking out dress sizes. Buy a pair of trousers one size down and try them on every couple of weeks – you'll notice that they get easier and easier to put on.
3. Seeing how much longer you can stay on the cross-trainer.
4. Being able to squeeze between cars in a car park without taking a wing mirror off.
5. Being able to walk down the aisle of an aeroplane without decapitating someone or having to walk sideways.
6. Noticing that your rings are now too big.

Saturday, 16 April 2005

Trevor arrived in London at 9 o'clock this evening and I really, really wanted a glass of vino – but it's only five-and-a-half weeks to 'reveal' day, so I didn't.

So desperate, though, that I had an Ally McBeal moment, which involved working out how I could drink wine without my friends stopping me. I fantasized about wrenching the bottle of wine out of Trevor's hands, knocking him out so that he couldn't stop me drinking, and then putting the wine on its side on the table and lying underneath it. Then, in my mind, I opened my mouth and drank the whole lot.

But I'm so close to 'reveal' day and I'm feeling so good about myself, that I can resist these temptations. I'm also really comfortable with the *You Are What You Eat* healthy eating now. I know exactly what to buy. I don't need to text Gillian so much any more. It's like when a bird flies the nest.

I trust myself now. I knew I'd have been all right with a glass of wine, but I still didn't betray that trust in myself. I'm glad I didn't do it. When I do start drinking again it's going to be so controlled. Partly because I'll kill myself if I drink more than a glass or two of wine on a night out. I won't have the tolerance now.

Monday, 18 April 2005

I love it. People are really starting to notice the difference in me.

I had a chat with Dax today and we spoke about stepping up the programme and increasing my sessions to three days a week, what with 'reveal' day being so close.

I came home in agony from the workout and made a delicious turkey dinner with my own sage-and-onion stuffing.

Turkey Stuffed with Sage and Onion

Turkey is extremely low in fat and therefore a great choice if you're trying to lose weight. It's also high in protein, B vitamins and selenium.

2 handfuls of fresh sage
1 tsp of red onion, peeled and chopped
1 garlic clove, peeled and chopped
1 tsp of extra virgin olive oil
1 turkey breast

Preheat the oven to 225°C, gas mark 7. Place the sage, onion, garlic and olive oil in a blender or food processor. Blend together for a minute or so to form a thick paste. Next, slice the turkey breast down the middle, so the halves are opened out but not separated. Fill the middle of the breast with the sage and onion stuffing, close up and then carefully wrap it in lightly oiled kitchen foil. Place in the oven and cook for 30 to 35 minutes. Serve with lots of steamed vegetables.

Tuesday, 19 April 2005

Oh my God, I'm on the front cover of *heat* magazine. How exciting. It was a very positive piece. They were lovely to me and it's really encouraging that people are still interested.

I had a meeting at 19 and Nicki Chapman advised me to eat less and jog more. I looked at her and thought, 'That's a really odd thing to say. I've lost four-and-a-half stone. Do you not think I know what I'm doing by now?' I felt a little weird after our chat. It was the first time I'd felt she was more interested in the public reaction than in me, which is wrong of me because she's not like that at all. It was just a throwaway comment. It wasn't meant to be taken personally.

I went to a Turkish restaurant with June for dinner and had hummus with crudités and falafel to start with and grilled chicken afterwards. I'm still keeping my carbs and my proteins separate, like a good girl.

It's just over a month to go now before we finish filming *You Are What You Eat*, and my flights to Spain are booked for the day after – 25 May. That's the week I'm focusing on.

Sunday, 24 April 2005

Dax is really turning up the heat. I was knackered after yesterday's workout.

Saw a delightful piece in the *Daily Star* today with a picture of me having a driving lesson. They assumed that I was only doing it now because I'd been too fat to get behind the wheel of a car before.

I went to a Japanese restaurant for lunch and had sea bass and miso soup. Japanese food is great because of all the fish, and because lots of the food contains the right type of fats.

SUPER SUSHI

Takeaways and junk food are not good for you. Full stop. But if you must have a 'fast fix', go for Japanese. The Japanese enjoy the best health and live the longest out of all the industrialized nations. Typical Japanese 'fast foods' like sushi and sashimi are very low in saturated fat – unlike the Western equivalents of burgers, kebabs or pizzas. They also provide essential fatty acids (EFAs), made up of omega-3 and omega-6 acids, which are necessary to maintain healthy skin, hair and bone tissue, to feed the brain and to help the body metabolize fats. EFAs stimulate weight reduction and also reduce cholesterol levels. Other goodies in the Japanese diet include ginger (see page 109), seaweed (see page 126) and miso soup (see page 124).

On the downside, a typical Japanese dish often contains soy sauce, which contains MSG, so don't over-season your sushi. Also, the rice is normally refined white rice, and as sushi usually contains both rice and fish, it breaks the rule of mixing carbs and protein. But once in a while, and if only to prevent a binge on junk food, sushi comes out tops.

Monday, 25 April 2005

My day of torture begins.

I start at 8 a.m. with a driving lesson, followed by a session with Dax Moy. Now I'm off to Margie for another colonic. Am I completely mad?

I was shattered after my session with Dax today. And I must call Gillian, because we haven't caught up with each other for a few weeks.

Wednesday, 27 April 2005

I saw Dax this morning and it's great news. In just one month, I have lost an inch from each arm, two inches from my waist, two inches from each thigh, and three-quarters of an inch from my bust – that last bit is not so good, actually, 'cos I love my boobs. Everything is coming together just in time for the show!

I'm having dinner with Laura's mate Ludwig tonight. He's flatmates with the guys from G4, the runners-up of *The X Factor* in 2004. I think G4 are really good. I saw *The X Factor* towards the end and I voted for them. Perhaps I liked them because they were the underdogs too. People say that *Pop Idol*, *Fame Academy* and *The X Factor* are shows to find gorgeous people who can sing, but I don't think that's what they're about. They have turned out to be for people like me and G4, who wouldn't get a record deal otherwise because we don't quite fit.

Unfortunately, Steve Brookstein, the winner of *The X Factor*, was dropped by his record company after only a few months – despite having over 5 million votes from fans. People who watch and vote on *Pop Idol* and *The X Factor* are not necessarily people who will turn those votes to sales by buying the music afterwards. Therefore, record companies need to know how to market to these people and make them buy records. The answer is simple: TV advertising and TV appearances to let people know you're still there. They need to market us reality-TV winners completely differently from the traditional pop star, because you have to go from TV star to serious musician in a short space of time. If they're going to get involved in reality TV they've got to understand what their end product will be and how to market it, because a crap, rushed album will flop and they'll be done for.

Thursday, 28 April 2005

What a nightmare: 19 have dropped me. I can't believe they would just do that with no warning. How ironic, given what I was writing about marketing reality-TV stars only yesterday. I contacted Ash – G4's manager – straight away, and he seemed really interested.

Maybe this is for the best. I've done all this hard work, losing weight and getting healthy, and they always knew I wanted to move on and do more music. However, after saying only a month ago, 'We're going to do this album and that single . . .' 19 are now claiming that they weren't ready to commit to another album.

I've been crying my eyes out. Now, looking and feeling as I do, I have my best chance ever of getting a record deal – but no management! I'm petrified. What's going to happen to me?

Friday, 29 April 2005

Things are beginning to look up. I've got a meeting on Wednesday with a PR guy, and my lawyer, Ann, has set up a few meetings with managers. Ash is just so busy with G4 that we'd be no good to each other at the moment. It would be like jumping from the frying pan into the fire.

This is a very vulnerable stage for me, and I realize I'm in danger of breaking my food regime: I've got no career, and no management. I'll just have to regroup quickly and become even more determined to lose weight – and to show them. It's especially important at times like this to stick to my lifestyle plan, and not to go into comfort-eating mode. In the past, that's exactly what I would have done.

Monday, 2 May 2005

I'm trying to forget career stuff, as it's a Bank Holiday, so I don't expect to hear anything from Ann today. I cooked one of my new favourite fish dishes for lunch.

Thursday, 5 May 2005

I spoke to Ann, who told me that manager and music guru Rick Blaskey really wants to talk to me, which is fantastic. We've booked a meeting for next Wednesday. I've sent him copies of all the magazines and newspapers I've been in over the past few weeks. I just want this to be sorted, as I feel very nervous. It's starting to occur to me for the first time that I might not make it as a recording artist. But if not that, then what? I'll exhaust all possibilities of getting a record deal first, and then I'll think.

It is an awful industry, though. And Mum and Dad get really heartbroken when things are written in the papers about me. When 'The Meaning Of Love' single bombed and went to

Fish with Pesto Crust

White fish is a good, low-calorie, low-fat source of protein, vitamins and minerals, and it therefore an ideal choice if you're trying to lose weight. Oily fish, such as salmon or mackerel, is a great source of omega-3 fatty acids.

2 handfuls of fresh basil
1 handful of pine nuts
1 garlic clove, peeled and crushed
1 tbsp of extra virgin olive oil
1 fillet of skinless and boneless fish – I use various different
    types of fish for this recipe, including salmon, halibut and
    sea bass
juice of half a lemon

Place the basil, pine nuts, garlic and oil in a blender or food processor. Blend together for a minute or so to make the pesto, then put it into a covered container and chill for 1 hour. Meanwhile, preheat the oven to 200°C, gas mark 6. Wrap the fish fillet into a parcel with kitchen foil, squeezing the lemon juice over the top of the fillet to prevent the foil from sticking. Spoon the chilled pesto over the top of the fish before closing up the parcel. Place in the oven and bake for 25 to 30 minutes. Serve with steamed vegetables.

Number 15, my dad and granddad came down to visit me and all the papers were saying I was finished. I didn't care. I knew I wasn't finished. My album had just got to Number 3.

But I could tell there was something not right about Dad. We were sitting in the back garden and Dad never drinks, because he can't handle too much, but he had two bottles of beer and burst out crying in front of eight or ten people because he couldn't take the worry. I had to hold my own dad and tell him it was OK and be really strong for him. Your parents love you so much that they take that kind of stuff personally. I gave him another beer and then put him to bed and he slept for eighteen hours.

But I can't stop here. I want to be in the music industry even though it's a nightmare. I thrive on it. I don't care whether the next album is a huge seller – I just want to feel that I've tried.

I'm very excited about tomorrow – I've been given a free weekend at the five-star Pennyhill Park spa in Surrey because of the health regime with Gillian, so I'm going with my sister Lynsey for my birthday weekend.

Saturday, 7 May 2005

This hotel is heaven. Had a fruit salad for breakfast, and now I'm off to the spa for a swim and various different treatments all afternoon.

I want to live here for ever. I've just had a full body exfoliation, then a mud wrap, followed by full body massage.

Gillian's just texted, telling me I was bossy because I told her to leave me alone this weekend. This is *my* weekend. It's been a stressful time recently and I need a break. She needn't be concerned, anyway. I don't eat when I worry!

Sunday, 8 May 2005

Twenty-five years old today and a size 18 – not bad.

I also weighed myself today, and I'm 17 stone 2 pounds. I've lost well over four-and-a-half stone!

I think this is my first sober birthday since I was fourteen. I'm not proud of that record. I started drinking when I was thirteen, the same way a lot of people do – standing outside shops, begging alcoholic tramps to buy us cider. And they would, because they could get us two bottles of cider and keep the change.

Wednesday, 11 May 2005

I've seen Dax every day for the last three days. The man's a god when it comes to fitness. Last session today for this week and I turned up an hour early. We did some boxing – I loved it.

Then I met Rick Blaskey and he blew me away. He's worked with Whitney Houston and represented Mica Paris. He reminds me of Dad as well, and I trust him to be the man to support me and respect the fact that I've put all this effort into changing my life.

If it doesn't work out I'll be back singing 'The Power Of Love' with Bessie up at the Blantyre Working-men's Club before long.

Monday, 16 May 2005

I just did a quick raid on Glasgow again. Flew up on Friday, packing my little lunch of carrot and hummus for the plane.

Everyone was so shocked at how I look. I love coming home, especially when people haven't seen me for a while.

This morning I did my exercises and packed my bags for my trip back to London. I slept all the way on the flight and didn't even eat the mung bean stew I made earlier. I don't really worship at the altar of the mung and the aduki – I'm not too keen on the taste – but I know from Gillian how good they are for me.

Wednesday, 18 May 2005

It's my last session with Dax before the show and my holiday. I'm free, I tell you, free!

I'm having a meeting with Faye, my stylist, later to work out what I'll be wearing for the 'reveal shot' at the end of the *You Are What You Eat* show.

Faye can't believe the difference in me. Last time she dressed me I was a size 26. I loved all the clothes she's picked.

Monday, 23 May 2005

I've just been to Ireland with Trevor for a wedding. Although they all know he's gay, no one's confirmed it so I went as his 'partner'. I looked amazing, if I do say so myself. I was wearing that dress again.

There were 350 at the sit-down meal alone – I had vegetable soup and grilled monkfish. Met a lovely guy called J. What a wedding. I was dying – it didn't finish until 5 a.m. and then we didn't sleep and I had to fly home yesterday.

Apparently, at 3 a.m. Trevor said, 'Where's Michelle?' and looked over to see me snogging the face off J.

Next up, sunny Spain and I'm so excited. This is what I've been working up to.

I got home and cleaned the house in preparation for the film crew arriving tomorrow. One day to alcohol.

Tuesday, 24 May 2005

16 stone 12 pounds

Oh my God, five months ago I was 21 stone 12 pounds.

I'm filming the last day of the first *You Are What You Eat* special today and I'm quite teary. Can't believe we got to the end of this first six months. I've really come to love filming days and it's strange to think it was only just a few months ago that I was crying in my house because I'd just been filmed in my swimsuit.

Today went fab. I celebrated with a glass of champers on the balcony and it tasted good.

Roll on Spain. The flight is booked for 1.40 p.m. from Stansted tomorrow.

Aaargh, just found out there's a bit of a problem: 19 are still doing my PR, and they've done an exclusive deal with *heat* magazine, which means *heat* have to be the first to get an opportunity to take pictures of me with my new slimline figure. If I go on holiday, people will take pics of me and we'll lose the deal with *heat*. So 19 are advising me not to go.

I don't think they realize what this holiday means to me. It's more than a holiday – it's a symbol. It's what I've worked towards. I didn't drink or sway from my healthy food, because all I'd thought about was this holiday. The holiday I'm flying out for tomorrow. After filming had wrapped, the whole point was to be that I left the very next day with all my girlfriends and I was going to get drunk and if I wanted to eat something I wasn't supposed to I could do so because it was my time. My chance to say, 'Well done, Michelle.'

Thank God, Nicki's made a compromise with *heat* magazine. Because *heat* want to shoot tomorrow, she says I can fly out afterwards if I agree not to go anywhere near the beach and risk a pap shot. I am going on the 25th, though. There's a flight at 5.30 p.m. which I'm sure I could catch. I don't want to miss a single day of this holiday.

Wednesday, 25 May 2005

I turned up for the *heat* shoot at 10 a.m. I had to get it done quickly as I really needed to make that flight. Spain was calling me.

Everyone was really relaxed, thinking we had a whole day to shoot in, and I was going 'Right!' like I was on *Changing Rooms*, straight in and out and getting loads done.

The shoot went fantastically well and I made it to Stansted in plenty of time.

Hola Spain! Touched down. I'm here.

Met the girls at the Hooper bar. And met up with a nice guy called S. He works out here.

Thursday, 26 May 2005

I'm loving Spain. But I'm sure I'm being punished for my drinking. I went out with Carrie till 7 a.m. – drinking with S –

and got mugged. We were walking past this bar literally a couple of yards from our apartment and a big group of ten Spanish guys came out. They started jumping all over us. We managed to fight them off, but as we walked to the apartment they backed us into the doors. There were only three of them by this point. The rest had run down the side of this restaurant and were shouting to the others to go – and they all disappeared.

Then suddenly I was hit on the head by my own bag, which now had nothing in it but the keys. I had been holding the kitty that night, and we had approximately 200–300 Euros between us, which was absolutely ridiculous. The guys had obviously got so much money out of us that they'd had a guilt trip and thought they'd better throw back our keys.

Then came the realization that we'd been robbed. We got in and woke everyone up, with Carrie saying, 'I've been mugged again!' She's already been mugged four times in Glasgow.

In my drunken state I tried to ring 999 and got some Spanish pizza takeaway instead. Back in the old days, I would have made the best of the situation and placed an order, but not now.

Friday, 27 May 2005

I'm dying. I can't cope with alcohol, and will be taking it so easy today. I stuck to white wine last night and must have had about seven glasses of it – which is just over a bottle. I'm definitely not going out tonight. Laura's going to make a nice salad, and I'm not drinking.

Gillian has been texting me – 'How are you coping?' – and so on. Don't know what to tell her.

ALCOHOL TO AVOID

1. Lager, beer, cider – the biggest bloaters of them all. They're full of bubbles, sugar and other crap
3. Alcopops – sugar city
4. Cream liqueur – cream: can't be good
5. Shots – they're deceptively small so you end up drinking more of them
6. Spirits with a gassy mixer like Coke – opt for fresh juice to go with it (or, my favourite: neat)
7. Cocktails – full of sugar

SENSIBLE DRINKING

There's no getting away from it – booze is an enemy of the healthy lifestyle (see page 76). Boo. But unless you're trying to lose a lot of weight, you can have the occasional drink on the *You Are What You Eat* plan. The main thing to remember is to stick well within the recommended limits of alcohol units per week, currently 21 units for men and 14 units for women. Remember that many pub measures are misleading – one 175ml glass of wine equals 2 units, for example, as does one pint of normal-strength lager. One 275ml bottle of alcopop has a value of 1.5 units. It's also important to include a number of alcohol-free days every week and to avoid binge drinking at all times. According to the Office of National Statistics, 36 per cent of men and 27 per cent of women in the 16–24 age group drink heavily at least once a week, defined as consuming eight or more units for men and six or more units for women in one night. Yet the health consequences can be devastating: severe liver damage, an increased risk of stroke, alcohol poisoning, not to mention the increased probability of being involved in an accident or a violent incident. If you are pregnant or likely to become pregnant, you should drink no more than one or two units a week, and it is safest to avoid alcohol altogether.

Nonetheless, there are times when a drink is welcome for all of us, so if you do fancy a tipple, which are the best and worst options to choose? Bubbly and gassy drinks cause bloating, and because beer and lager are often drunk in pints, you end up consuming a larger amount of liquid. So they're probably among the worst choices for dieters. On balance, a glass of red wine is probably the best drink for you as it contains antioxidants. And if you prefer spirits, vodka is perhaps the best in terms of calories and bloating; it's only about 50 calories a shot, is quite pure, not too sugary and doesn't contain yeast from fermentation. Gin's OK too, and white rum. Stick to fruit-juice mixers – freshly squeezed if possible – and always have lots of ice, as it will help to stop dehydration. Dehydration is one of the main factors that cause a hangover (though not the only one).

Other sensible tips to remember when you drink are to eat before you go out, drink slowly, alternate alcoholic drinks with glasses of water, and don't mix your booze. Obviously all this sensible advice went out the window as soon as I was on holiday . . .

Sunday, 29 May 2005

I went to Donna's house yesterday for a barbecue with the girls. There was always going to be trouble, as she makes a mean champagne sangria . . .

Donna's Mean Champagne Sangria

This is strictly only allowed as a special treat, and usually only on holiday, but it's soooooooooo delicious I had to put it in!

1 egg cup of brandy
2 egg cups of Cointreau
3 tbsp sugar
chopped fruit (melon, strawberries, and so on)
1 bottle of champagne (or, if no one is looking, cava)
lots of ice

Pour the brandy, Cointreau and sugar into a big sangria jug and mix together. Then add the fruit. Pour in a third of a bottle of champagne and stir until all the froth disappears, then continue pouring in the remainder of the champagne slowly, stirring all the while. Once all the bottle is in, add ice to fill up to the top of the jug and then stir again. Leave for a few minutes to settle, then serve.
   And don't tell Gillian.

Everyone's useless today and we went back to Donna's house to lie by the pool – because I can't go to the beach, obviously, due to the *heat* deal.

I'm being pretty good, though: one night on, two nights off. It's not exactly Gillian's 80:20 rule (more like 30:70), but hey, I'm on holiday.

Wednesday, 1 June 2005

Well, I did it! I pulled the lovely S last night. And it was worth playing hard to get and waiting a whole week. Just before going home, too.

Later, I texted him, saying, 'You're so dead, feeding me full of sambuca.'

Thursday, 2 June 2005

Back in London. I got a text from S: 'Lying on the beach with no hangover as I didn't touch a drop of sambuca and it feels great! How is London today?'

I'm going to the gym because I need to get straight back into the old routine now I'm back home.

Actually, somehow I lost 3 pounds on holiday. I did eat healthily and was quite active, I suppose. I'd planned to go absolutely nuts, but I just can't do it any more. My body had got used to large quantities of alcohol before I was on the *You Are What You Eat* plan so I could drink much more, but now I'm screwed – no tolerance!

Friday, 3 June 2005

I'm flying out to Glasgow again tonight as Carrie and I are going to a friend's engagement party tomorrow night.

And I'm back on my healthy-eating plan with no alcohol. I want to shed the rest of this weight a.s.a.p., so I'm a size 14. It shouldn't take much longer.

Monday, 20 June 2005

Whoops, left my diary in Scotland, which is why I haven't written for a while. I'm back in London now, though, and am doing an interview on the Fred MacAulay show today; he's a DJ on Radio Scotland. He was really supportive, saying, 'Good on you for doing this. We think you look great.' It's the first radio show I've done to promote the first *You Are What You Eat* show (which is going out on Channel 4 the day after tomorrow!) and I'm so relieved I seem to be getting a positive reaction. I thought people would be saying, 'Why have you done it? Why have you sold out?'

I went straight to Celador afterwards with a few people from 19, and we all watched the show for the first time. Oh my God – I love it. I can't believe that I've done this. It was such an emotional journey.

When I first came on and I saw what size I'd been, I couldn't breathe. I thought, 'I can't let people see me like this.' By the end, and the reveal shot, I just looked so different.

19 have also organized for me to appear on a new BBC show called *Departure Lounge*, as one of the guest presenters for their £500 challenge. It's a feature where you have to try to travel as far as possible and experience as many things for up to three days on a limited budget. Nicki Chapman's doing it and suggested I should, too – and where would I like to go? I said how about something to do with music?

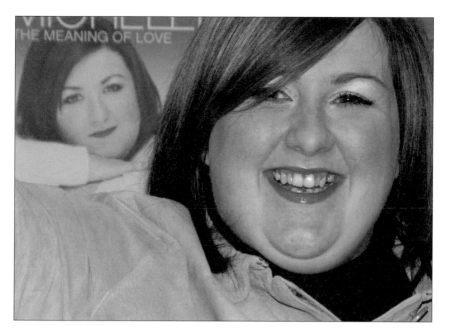

Promoting my debut album, *The Meaning of Love*, in February 2004. Post-*Pop Idol*, I was always on the road, and my eating habits proved catastrophic: I gained another three stone.

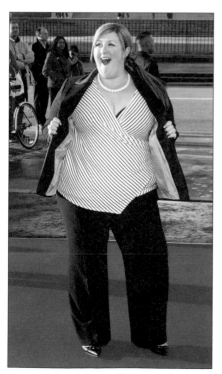

At 19 Management's nineteenth birthday party in April 2004. A year later, I would be leaving them for pastures new.

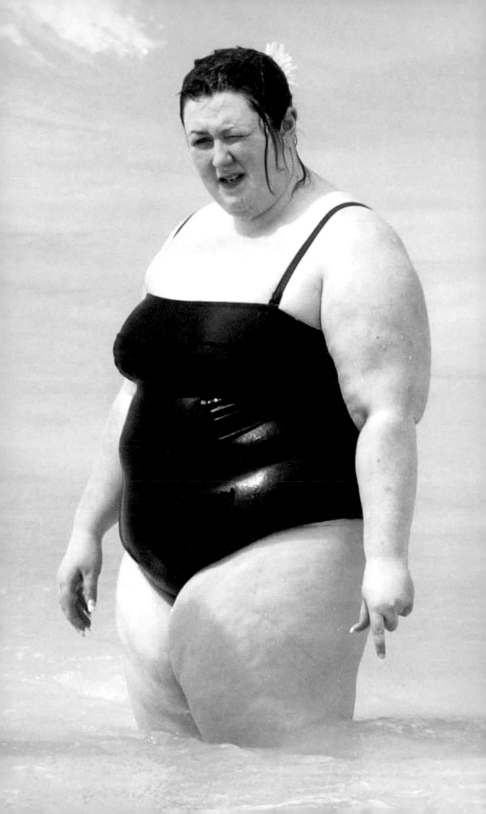

OPPOSITE PAGE: On the beach in Barbados in May 2004. I was so mortified when these pictures came out. In August that year, I was horrified to learn that my weight had crept up to 22 stone.

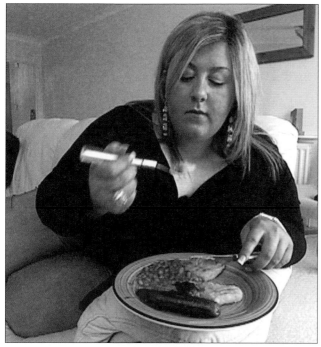

A typical breakfast before Gillian McKeith came into my life.

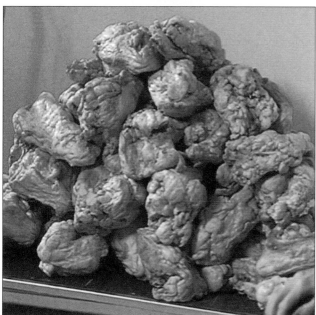

Of the entire *You Are What You Eat* programme, the most difficult moment was when I was presented with 11.5 stone of animal fat to show me my excess weight. It was disgusting.

Getting to grips with my new healthy eating regime. Unbelievably, I'm now a devotee of colonics, too – though I don't look entirely comfortable here! (*below right*)

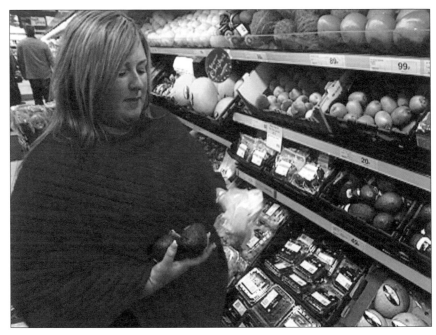

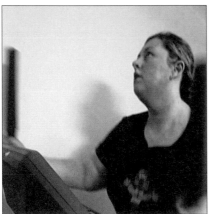

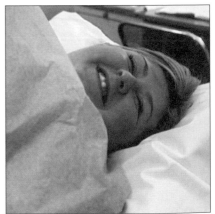

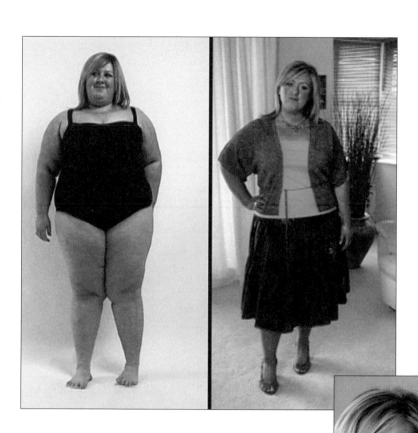

SPOT THE DIFFERENCE: From fat to fantastic in the time it takes to lose five-and-a-half stone. This is me before and after the first *You Are What You Eat* programme, six months into the plan.

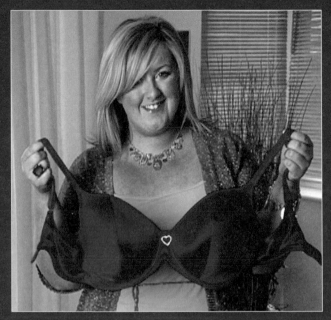

Me with an old bra. Dropping five dress sizes has meant a whole new wardrobe for me ... well, any excuse to go shopping!

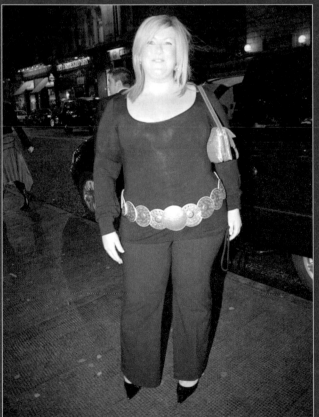

FILTHY GORGEOUS: At the *Goal!* premiere in September 2005, looking and feeling great.

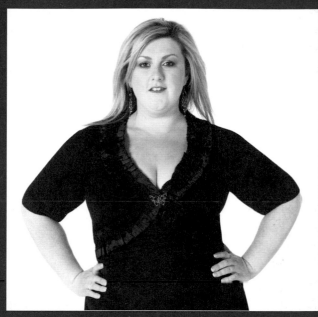

Christmas 2005.
The new me!

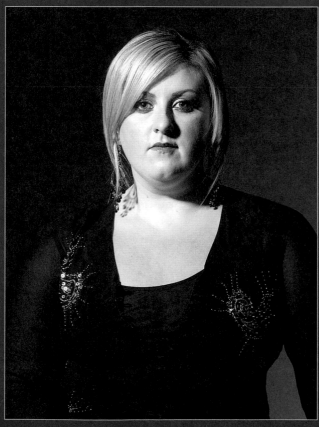

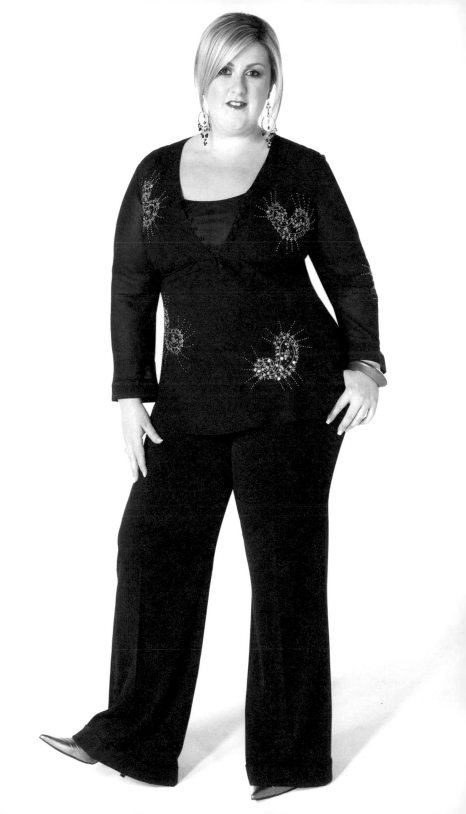

How about Elvis's home in Memphis, Graceland? They loved the idea.

Tuesday, 21 June 2005

I'm doing a radio interview on the telephone with Irish radio station Beat 102–103. I love doing promo in Ireland. Everyone is so friendly and it reminds me of being back home. I'm getting really, really nervous about tomorrow, though – the public transmission date for the first *You Are What You Eat* special. Then again, I'm proud of it, and what's done is done.

I was also interviewed on Richard and Judy's show today. They were so lovely. I had to share a dressing room with Gillian; she was there to talk about her recipe book. 'You've got to plug the book because all your recipes are in there,' she told me. I replied, 'Plug your own book!'

David Schwimmer from *Friends* was also there, because he's starring in *Some Girls* in the West End. Gillian and I were pressed up against the window of his dressing room trying to see him. Then G said, 'I'm just going to go out and talk to him.' She's so brazen like that. But he was in the middle of being interviewed by Jamie Theakston for Jamie's radio show.

I was all glammed up and they were really interested in talking about me rather than Gillian. But Gillian and I can have a laugh together. She was saying, 'Richard, did I tell you about my book?' At that point Richard was trying to interview me, and I said, 'By the way, does everyone know that Gillian's got a book out? Can everyone just go and buy it?' Richard was killing himself laughing.

He also said, 'Something really strange has happened with

your breasts. They went from 46DD to a 38G. How very odd!' It's true, although I've no idea how he knew that. I've lost four inches off my waist and three-and-a-half inches from each thigh, and my bust has increased in cup size, but decreased in back size! Rigby & Peller were baffled.

I'd never met Richard and Judy before, and I didn't know what they thought of me and what I'd done. Richard's notorious for being a bit of a loose cannon, and I thought he might say, 'Why say you're happy and then do this?' But they were both really lovely and among the nicest interviewers I've ever spoken to.

It's an early night for me tonight, because I'm up at 4.30 tomorrow morning for *GMTV* – with Gillian again.

Wednesday, 22 June 2005

The big day.

I woke up at 4.30 a.m. – and I'm cacking myself now. Oh God. What if people think I'm an idiot?

I really want people to understand why I did this, but then again, why do I care so much what other people think?

I did *GMTV* this morning with Ben Shepherd and Fiona Phillips. Ben Shepherd's interviewed me a couple of times before and he was like, 'God, you look amazing.' They're such lovely people, they really are. Fiona came and spoke to me while I was getting my make-up done, telling me, 'Well done for doing it,' and 'You're such an inspiration.'

I was also interviewed by Lorraine Kelly, who's a fellow Scot, so we were all speaking the same language. It was so funny. Between us we teased Gillian lots, but Gillian took it really well. All day today friends and family have been talking about what a fab show it was with Lorraine. She's so sweet.

Then it was straight to *Reveal* magazine for a photo shoot, as I'm doing a big story with them. Right in the middle of the shoot there was a call from *Channel 4 News*! Obesity figures were published today and there have been calls to ban junk-food advertisements on TV. Jon Snow and the team asked if I would go on and talk about how I got so overweight and whether junk-food advertising had affected me.

Initially I didn't want to appear on the programme, but then I thought, 'How many pop stars are asked to go on *Channel 4 News*? I can't say no.' After all, I told myself, I'm not a doctor but I can hold my own. If they ask me questions, I'm just going to give them my opinion.

As it turns out, it was a great success and they've asked me to come back in the future. And Jon Snow! I actually fell in love with Jon Snow. He said, 'What an honour to meet you. My daughters love you. Can I just say what a pleasure it is to have you on the show?' I was just thinking, 'You're . . . J-J-J-Jon . . . S-S-S-Snow.' I love *Channel 4 News*. It's real broadsheet, hard-hitting news and they've got me at the beginning of the show, live from the make-up room!

He asked whether I thought junk-food advertisements had contributed to me being overweight and I replied, 'No, I genuinely don't think it did. I don't remember looking at an ad and thinking, "Must go and buy a McDonald's." I was just a child of the junk-food age and I got a real taste for it. The reason I became overweight was that I didn't eat healthily and I didn't exercise. I don't have a thyroid problem. I'm not big-boned. There's nothing wrong with me.'

When he asked how I lost the weight, I told him that I just ate healthily and exercised, simple as that. Afterwards, he said he loved my directness. I guess it's a relief after all those politicians. And people love to hear from real people who've lost weight and changed themselves.

I went straight home and watched the transmission of *You Are What You Eat* with my mates and cried again. Received a million calls and took part in a web-chat. A couple of thousand people were waiting to speak to me!

It's been a very, very surreal day, but one of the best days of my life.

Thursday, 23 June 2005

Well, Celador are over the moon with the show: it had 3.8 million viewers and peaked at 4.6 million – the highest they've ever had by far (they usually get somewhere between 3 and 4 million). They defo want to do a second show, but I need to get things sorted with 19 first.

Everyone's talking about the show!

Friday, 24 June 2005

To the gym, then for a swim, and then to get my hair done because it's my friend Barney's Big Birthday tonight.

I had a good night but didn't drink, as I want to drink next weekend when I see all my friends in Bristol and go to a charity ball – so my plan is to stay sober till then. Check out me and my new-found self-control and respect for my body! I can't drink like I used to and I don't want to build my tolerance up again, because unfortunately, if you want to lose weight, you have to cut alcohol out or cut it right down. I'm so comfortable with drinking rarely now, and feel much better for drinking in moderation.

I wonder whether Gillian's going to freak when she finds out that I've drunk anything at all, but my attitude is that I've been doing this for so many months now that my life has got to go back to some sort of normality sooner or later. I'm still taking my own food everywhere with me, and I'm exercising. And I'm at a weight and stage where I'm happy to have the occasional glass of wine. I probably only drink a couple of times a month now. I know what she's going to say, but tough.

Sam from *Pop Idol* was out and it was nice to see him.

Sunday, 26 June 2005

Yesterday I was up at 8 a.m. to clean the house because my sisters were coming down. We had a good night, but I stayed sober. Ludwig, Laura's mate, took the girls back to his flat and gave them scones and jam with cream. Gay men – love 'em. Only Ludwig would have clotted cream and jam at his flat. I had a banana.

Went to the organic supermarket Fresh & Wild to buy lunch. My sisters hate coming to stay with me because there's no food in the house they want to eat – no milk, no white bread – and even when we eat out I still insist on health food. If they want a cup of tea there are teabags but no milk, as I'm still avoiding cow's milk. Or I'll go and buy a loaf of bread so they can have toast, then get back and realize there's no butter.

'How about a packet of crisps?'
'I don't keep crisps.'

I've forgotten how other people eat. Actually, my sisters eat fairly healthily – Caesar salad, pasta with tomato sauce – but Gillian would no doubt say they ate like animals.

In the old days I'd have had a 24-pack of crisps in the cupboard, big bottles of Diet Coke in the fridge and as many microwave meals and pizzas as I could cram into the freezer.

Monday, 27 June 2005

I did a photo shoot today for *Simply Be* (a plus-size catalogue) in aid of breast cancer research. It was a great laugh. *Simply Be* is amazing and they've just joined with Anna Scholz, who's one of my favourite designers for big women. A jacket by her would have cost £500 or £600 from Selfridges, but now she's doing an affordable range for bigger women, and for younger women who are bigger. Next and Dorothy Perkins are also good and go up to a size 20. But it's still really rare for designers to cater for larger women. I don't think a lot of designer labels want their clothes on bigger girls. Also, I've heard from my friend, who's a buyer for a clothes store in Glasgow, that there's no demand for them – that bigger women don't want to wear designer labels. I wonder if that's really true and, if so, why? Maybe it's a self-esteem thing.

Tuesday, 28 June 2005

My sisters Maria and Lynsey went home today. We went to the little French restaurant down the road first and had salad for lunch. They had spritzers and I had water. I was really tempted to drink, but decided against it. Can't go back to my wicked ways full time.

I'll be chilling out tonight and doing my exercises.

Wednesday, 29 June 2005

I now love swimming – and it's amazing how much fitter I am than six months ago.

Went to the hairdresser's afterwards, as tonight I have a dinner date with Gillian McKeith. She's taking me out to celebrate the success of the show.

We went to Gordon Ramsay's restaurant near Hyde Park Corner and Gillian practically ordered my entire meal for me. Had veggie soup to start, followed by monkfish, which was supposed to come with mashed potato and cream sauce – but Gillian asked them to change the mash and cream sauce. She's much more confident than I am about ordering off-menu.

Although I've got a good idea of what I can eat now, re-educating myself has taken time. I needed that initial six months under Gillian's close supervision and I'm still learning about food now, but I'm in the swing of things. I can't remember not knowing what to eat. Now I can go into a health-food shop, look at the back of a nut bar that claims to be all natural and know what to look out for – if it contains E numbers or sodium then I won't touch that bar.

I'm still not allowed to drink as far as Gillian's concerned, but I have treated myself to the odd tipple. I'm so deeply into this new healthy lifestyle that I think I can allow myself that, because nothing's going to knock me out of it. Nine out of ten times I still won't drink, though.

But although I know I can drink occasionally and not put weight on, I find I don't always want it any more. I don't crave it like I did during the first six months. And if I do go out and have a few, I'll wake up the next day and have a smoothie, a banana and then a big plate of goat's cheese salad, because there's nothing better for a hangover and it's quite stodgy enough for me now. There's no need for a fry-up any more.

Gillian told me that when we first met at the offices of 19 and Nicki had said Gillian liked me, Gillian herself had actually stormed out of the meeting saying it wasn't going to work. She said that I didn't have the right attitude and that I was going to fail, adding, 'I'm not willing to put my name to this because I've never failed before.' But Celador had told her, 'She's a really lovely girl, honestly. She really wants to work with you.'

I told Gillian about how I'd instantly hated her and wanted to put her through a window, and how I'd thought, 'Right, I'll show you what I can do,' because she obviously had no faith in me.

Of course, that was actually her game plan. She'd said months before that she was dying to work with me. She laughed when I pointed that out. That's what I like about her.

Thursday, 30 June 2005

I started doing a bit of kickboxing with Dax Moy this morning, and loved it. It gives you a fab shape, but it kills when you're doing it.

Friday, 1 July 2005

Swimming today and then off to see Rick Blaskey. Lovely man. We spoke about future plans and album deals etc., and it was all very positive. We've arranged with Celador to discuss the next show.

Saturday, 2 July 2005

The weekend I've been saving myself for. I haven't had any alcohol since Spain, five weeks ago, but I'd decided I was going to allow myself to go for it a bit with my friends in Bristol at tonight's charity ball.

I got up very early and went to the hairdresser's with June, and then started off for Bristol and the ball. Picked up Vikki and headed straight for the hotel. As it turned out, I had a fab night. I'd taken along some Rachel Stevens and Will Young CDs from 19 and they raised quite a bit of money.

And I was bought for £120 – for a kiss, anyway. I even pulled a Chris Martin lookalike!

I am much more confident about my body now. I don't look in the mirror and see a fat girl any more – I just see a big girl with hips and a bum and a belly. And I feel easier about pulling now because I feel more like someone should want to pull me. I think, 'You're so lucky for coming over to talk to me and you don't even know it yet.'

It's not just about looking good and feeling good; it's about being proud of yourself for what you've achieved.

PULLING FOODS

Gillian has explained to me how the food we eat and our sex lives are inextricably linked. The right foods can enhance sexual potency, make you feel more up for it and, if you're a woman trying to get pregnant, help with fertility. A lack of good foods can slow your sex drive, however. Some food she recommends for good sex includes avocados, blueberries, garlic (surprise!), mangoes, oats, spinach and watercress. Not sure about putting them all together, though.

Sunday, 3 July 2005

I didn't feel that drunk last night, but now I have the most horrendous hangover. It might be because I pulled and haven't been to sleep. I only had four glasses of wine, but it feels like five bottles. The truth is, I can't handle my drink any more. Whatever happened to Michelle 'Oddbins' McManus?

My plan of action today is to go for a healthy walk and then die in silence.

In pain. In pain.

Monday, 4 July 2005

How wonderful not to wake up with a hangover. Even if it is at 5 a.m. June's decided to drive back to London this morning. She's a nutcase. I've decided to sleep all the way in the car.

Tuesday, 5 July 2005

Off to the gym. This time I did a workout and then went swimming.

I went to Clapham Junction to collect my ball gown from the dry-cleaner's and get some food in. That's the only problem with this *You Are What You Eat* thing – you go shopping, come out with seventeen heavy bags of fruit and veg, and then have to try to get on a packed bus with them.

Wednesday, 6 July 2005

I had my last driving lesson today – the test is tomorrow. I really, really hope I pass, but I'm totally prepared to fail too.

I'm so excited: I've got a styling meeting with *InStyle* magazine this afternoon. They're doing a body issue and they want me to take part as I am now a beautiful size 18!

Thursday, 7 July 2005

London is in a total mess. There have been four bombs on tubes and buses. Lots of people have been killed and injured.

Failed my driving test, but who cares? There are more important things going on in the world at the moment.

I weighed myself and I am still 16 stone 11 pounds, so

I've stayed the same weight for six weeks. I guess my body's stabilizing.

Friday, 8 July 2005

I tried on some skirts today that fitted me about six weeks ago, but are now really loose.

That said, my weight has plateaued. Although I'm getting slimmer in terms of dress sizes, when I step on the scales I weigh the same as I have for the last six weeks. Maybe it's because I completely body-swerved the daily meditations that Gillian recommended me to do every morning all those months ago.

It's funny, though, how some things I used to be sceptical about I'm now much more convinced by. For example, food combining – the 'don't combine protein and carbs' rule. In a way this was easier for me. Because I was trying to lose a lot of weight, I was told to steer clear of the kinds of things you usually combine with proteins anyway, like potatoes (no jacket potato with tuna), bread (no chicken sandwiches), and white rice. So it wasn't that much of a struggle to keep the groups separate.

Also, I really believe now that calories aren't the most important thing when it comes to losing weight. For example, even though I'm 'on a diet', I probably still eat 2,000 calories a day. For a snack I might eat a packet of mini-carrots and a whole tub of hummus, which is 600 calories but only contains chickpeas, water, tahini (which is sesame-seed pulp), lemon juice and garlic. That's it. If you eat more calories than you use you will gain weight, but with a healthy lifestyle it's actually hard to eat too many calories, especially if you're opting for lots of fresh fruit and vegetables, which fill you up without adding lots of fat to your diet. The important thing is to eat lots of wholesome, nutritious food, and not starve yourself in the name of healthy eating.

Saturday, 9 July 2005

I got up this morning and made my guests, Anne and Wayne, a fry-up, but when they saw my lovely breakfast of fruit they requested the healthy option tomorrow. I'm having an effect on them!

Went to see *The Producers* and had one glass of white wine. I was legless.

Sunday, 10 July 2005

I woke up and made everyone a healthy breakfast of juice and fruit and we ate on the balcony, overlooking the river. It's days like this that I love my new eating habits, especially when others join in.

Having said that, I went to the Ship Inn in Wandsworth for lunch with friends and I could have murdered a beer. The weather was beautiful – this is definitely drinking weather. Everyone had lovely big pints of lager. I used to love lager, but that and Jack Daniel's and Coke are the two things, hand on my heart, that I haven't touched since the beginning of the *You Are What You Eat* plan. Lager's a whole different ball game. I'd be scared of what I'd do to myself – all the bloating and everything.

Wednesday, 13 July 2005

I went to see Rick Blaskey today as things are really starting to move with the management deal. Fingers crossed with the record deal now.

Back to Battersea Park and I lay out in the sun reading for four hours. Did the same thing a couple of days ago after a great day's shopping – found out that I'm buying some size 16s now. It's amazing.

Thursday, 14 July 2005

I had my first day back filming with *You Are What You Eat* again for their second special, which is going to come out in December. It was quite weird. We shot as if I'd just watched the programme and we did a post-show interview on my thoughts and feelings about the six months to come. I just went on about maintaining a healthy lifestyle and not putting on weight.

I suppose I'm scared that:

a) I won't lose any more weight, and
b) I'll start to put weight back on.

I just need to be really strong and keep going, as I have at least another couple of stone to lose before Christmas.

It was strange filming without 19, though.

Tuesday, 19 July 2005

A barbecue last night at June's. I took along a great barbecue recipe that everyone wanted to try.

Tuna and Salmon Kebabs

(serves 4)

Proof that you can have a good, old-fashioned barbie and still eat healthily! No need to load up on sausages and burgers – these kebabs are full of those omega-3 fatty acids, and taste delicious.

2 tuna steaks
2 salmon fillets
2 onions, cut into large pieces
8 cherry tomatoes
juice of 1 lemon

Chop the steaks of tuna and salmon into chunks, and thread them onto kebab skewers, alternating them with the pieces of raw onion and cherry tomatoes. Pour the lemon juice over and place on a hot barbecue for 5 to 10 minutes, turning regularly so that they cook evenly.

Wednesday, 20 July 2005

Went swimming today and then to see my accountants to talk about life after 19. We also discussed how I should stop my spending from going out of control. For anyone who thinks they just need a bit more money to solve all their problems, that's crap. You'll still overspend. The more money you have the more you'll spend – simple as that.

Weighed myself and I'm 16 stone 7 pounds – whooo-hooo! I've lost 5 pounds in a couple of weeks.

Friday, 22 July 2005

Busy, busy day. Styling meeting in Harrods with *InStyle* magazine. Oh my God, the clothes I'm going to be modelling are beautiful. I've never looked so sexy.

It was the first episode of *Extras* on the telly last night. I loved it. I really fancy Ricky Gervais. I met him at Teddington Studios in September 2003 when I was down to the last fifty in *Pop Idol*. It was in the old days and I was suffering greatly because I'd been hammered the night before and I was telling him all my drunken stories. He was killing himself laughing. I was thinking, 'Is Ricky Gervais laughing at *me*?' I was nicknamed 'Oddbins' by Kate Thornton because the party was always back in my room. I was dead worried at the time because I had such a huge room bill and I didn't think my credit card was going to work, and he thought it was hilarious.

Sunday, 24 July 2005

Such an exciting day. I went to do *Big Brother's Little Brother* and then I was given a tour of the *Big Brother* house. I know it's sad, but I love it. And I jumped at the chance because I adore Dermot O'Leary.

It was amazing. We were so well treated. Dermot was just as lovely as you'd expect. I did wonder whether they really wanted to hear my opinions though, because I'm just some reality-TV star. I went to Livebait's Café Fish in Soho afterwards with my friend Barney to thank him for getting me the gig on *BBLB* – he was a researcher on it last year. Bought a bottle of wine, but couldn't touch it. Barney drank the whole bottle instead.

Monday, 25 July 2005

Doing an interview with *Channel Five News* regarding the new, so-called 'diet jab' today. It's a self-administered dose of a naturally occurring hormone that's meant to make you want to eat less.

I said anything that can help people can only be a good thing, but that it's not something I would consider because what would I learn by injecting myself? Nothing. I'd still eat the same crap. I went on to say that the only reason this regime has worked for me is because I've actually taken the time to completely re-educate myself.

Then this afternoon it was the *InStyle* photo shoot. This is the most exciting photo shoot ever. They've made me look so beautiful. They dressed me in the designer vintage clothing we discussed at the styling meeting, and gave me beautiful blonde hair extensions. I wore a satin vintage opera coat with a big, wide Japanese belt around it, and six-and-a-half-inch YSL heels that I could only stand in for short periods of time. The photographer was really complimentary. He was saying, 'You look really sexy. I'd buy that outfit if I were you.'

Of course I did – any man saying I look sexy is good enough for me.

Got home and collapsed in bed with a herbal tea.

MY TOP TEN TEAS

1. Nettle – tasty to my newly clean palate and supposed to help general health too
2. Fennel – meant to be good for settling the stomach after a meal
3. Peppermint – again good for digestion, so another excellent alternative to the after-lunch coffee
4. Camomile – makes you sleepy and calm, so good in the evening
5. Ginger and lemon – helps digestion (the ginger) and has soothing, even antiseptic properties (the lemon)
6. Strawberry – tasty, and settles and cleanses the stomach
7. Blackcurrant – traditionally a soother of the throat, but tastes great too
8. Apple and cinnamon – said by some to cleanse and balance the system
9. Orange and mango – supposed to settle the stomach and sweeten the breath
10. Raspberry and loganberry – raspberry is refreshing and also a gentle laxative if you're feeling blocked up

I'm feeling really thin for me at the moment. Weighed myself: 16 stone 3 pounds.

Looking forward to going to Ireland on Thursday. And I'll be seeing J again soon – the guy I pulled at the wedding last time I was in the Emerald Isle.

Saturday, 30 July 2005

Arrived in Dublin yesterday.

I'm starting to get very nervous about meeting J tonight, as we have been texting for two months. Well, I look fab, so here goes. I hope he's as nice as I remember.

Sunday, 31 July 2005

What a bloody disaster.

J and I were having a great time, then when we went outside, he got this phone call. He started really arguing with this person over the phone, and it sounded like a woman. He was saying, 'No, no. I'm not out. I'm not doing anything.' I was like, 'Hmm. He was definitely single at the wedding.'

Then he said, 'Give me two minutes,' and disappeared down an alley.

After five minutes I thought, 'I'd better go and check that he's OK.' So I walked down the alleyway only to find that he'd gone. Just disappeared. And this from a guy who during the last couple of months has sent me over 500 text messages. Maybe he thinks I'm playing with him. He was really freaked out to see me on the front cover of *heat* magazine. Men!

Tuesday, 9 August 2005

Had a midday meeting with Phyllis Walters regarding going to Milan to support the plus-size catwalk shows. She's in fashion PR and represents Elena Mirò, which is an Italian fashion house that makes clothes from size 14 to 20. They're looking for somebody around a size 16 to promote their clothing, so she called me for a meeting, which is quite cool.

Then at 3 p.m. I had a meeting with Emma (researcher) and Ed (director) regarding my trip to Memphis and Graceland for *Departure Lounge*.

While I was sitting in the pub for the meeting, this absolutely gorgeous Portuguese guy came up to me and tried to buy me a drink. I didn't know how to deal with it because I was in company and this never happens to me normally. As I was about to leave he ran over.

'Are you going to give me your phone number?' he asked.

'No.'

'Well, can I give you mine then? Honestly, I used to be twenty stone myself and I watched you on *You Are What You Eat*. I thought you were beautiful anyway, but I think you're beautiful now and I really fancy you.'

This guy must have lost shedloads of weight. But I would never phone him because he might be a journalist, he might be anyone. I don't trust people since winning *Pop Idol*. It's not only that I've had bad experiences, but you just don't know who anyone is and they know all about you – they know your star sign, your favourite food, your dog's name when you were growing up. It's bizarre. After winning the show I remember one time when I got chatting to this really nice guy at a bar, and after an hour or so he said, 'I hate to tell you this, but I'm actually from the *Sun* newspaper.'

I just looked at him and said, 'What?' I was almost in tears.

He kept it going for another couple of minutes and then said, 'I'm kidding.' I just walked away.

Thursday, 11 August 2005

Very excited. I arrived at Gatwick this morning for the filming of *Departure Lounge* and was met by the crew. Vanessa Feltz was also there, as she is doing a challenge too. She was lovely – and another lady who's done wonders losing weight.

I got upgraded to first class by sticking a camera in the face of the check-in person and – oh my God – I don't think I can ever fly economy again. The seats are like double beds. You get an à la carte menu to choose from instead of the usual microwaved, stinking, salt-infested airline food. It was luxury. There was also champagne, though I didn't drink it.

Oh God, it's 12.30 a.m. Memphis time, which means it's 6.30 a.m. UK time. I've been up for twenty-four hours.

Friday, 12 August 2005

Woke up at 5.30 a.m. Can't sleep. Jet-lagged.

Took the Greyhound bus to Clarksdale, Mississippi. We went to the Delta Blues festival, a celebration of blues music that's been going for nearly thirty years. It lasts for two days and acts come from all over America to perform. The talent is just unbelievable.

I'm finding it really, really tough to eat healthily here. It's worse than Glasgow for deep-fried food. I asked for some grilled chicken and I swear it was fried. I don't know what I'm going to do. I really don't want to eat badly, having got this far.

It's going to be 40 degrees tomorrow.

No word from J.

Saturday, 13 August 2005

I got up and left Uncle Ben's Hotel – where Tennessee Williams used to stay – at 8.30 a.m. and headed out for breakfast. The director was a bit of a pain. He knows I need to eat healthily, but he took us to a roadside café that served fried breakfasts. I asked them if they had fruit and the woman thought I was nuts; I had to go to a supermarket to buy some.

Went to Graceland – whoa! Met Jerry Schilling, Elvis's best friend – whoa!

There's hope yet. Found a great place to eat called Café Francisco that did a fab Greek salad. Also went to Sun Studios and B.B. King's nightclub.

It's like nothing on earth to be here. I'm a size 16 and compared to the some of the women here I'm like a supermodel. And it's no wonder. The diet is atrocious. Even in the old days I think I'd have struggled to eat here. Everything's deep-fried. I don't know how the men do it – they look relatively normal.

Sunday, 14 August 2005

It's my last day and my stomach is in agony from lack of health food – in fact, lack of any food. I'm completely bunged-up and definitely need another colonic. Yesterday I was starving, so I got this harmless-looking white vegetable wrap. I'm in torture now because I've eaten white bread. It just ripped through my stomach. My body's got so used to eating wholegrains that it can't cope with processed white carbs now.

It's a shock because on the whole my poos don't smell any more since I've been eating healthily. If I eat dodgy stuff I know about it because I get an upset stomach the next day.

Tried to get first class again on the way back, but no chance. Bitch. 'No, honey. You don't pay for first class, you don't get first class.' This will be a long night and I refuse to eat any plane food. It's full of crap.

J texted me saying, 'Once and for all, let's get this sorted. I've got a perfectly good explanation. Give me a call and we'll sort this out.' I answered saying, 'Fine. Phone me, only because my curiosity's killing me and I want to know exactly what happened to you.'

Tuesday, 16 August 2005

I woke up, went to the gym and did a very intensive workout. Well-needed, too. I also spoke to Gillian, who was on top form.

Weighed myself and I've lost 2 pounds, but I'm feeling down. Simon Cowell trashed me in the *Daily Record* today. He said I was over and he only supported me during *Pop Idol* because there was no one else to support. I know that's not how he feels, it's just that he's got a new show coming up and it's all publicity for him. It still hurts, though.

Wednesday, 17 August 2005

Dental appointment with the hygienist today. If I'm going to look good, my teeth may as well look good too, even if they are a little bit crooked.

The *Sun* ran the Simon Cowell story. Bollocks.

I found out from Trevor that, in fact, J has a girlfriend. Why should I be surprised? He's a man. Texted him and told him not to contact me again.

Friday, 19 August 2005

Yesterday, after much indecision, I bought myself a tent for the V Festival at Chelmsford. Wasn't sure whether to stay in a hotel or to camp. I've not camped before. As a family we always used to go and stay in the Sea Inn at Morecambe Bay and we loved it. We saw Russ Abbot and people like that. It was a great time.

God alone knows how I'm going to build this tent. June begged for us to camp because I'd got VIP tickets and now we're going to be in the VIP camping area.

Had my first beetroot juice in ages. It tasted amazing and reminded me of my first few weeks of the *You Are What You Eat* lifestyle plan, which gave me a real boost. How far I've come. I'm so proud of myself. The beetroot drink is gorgeous, but for some reason I haven't been back to it for a while.

I bought a pair of boots in Primark for £12 – bargain. Also, bought all my fruit and veg for the festival and a cool box.

Saturday, 20 August 2005

Got to the festival and had to queue for an hour to get into the campsite. Finally made it in with my cool box laden with six pittas, two big salmon salads, loads of fruit and a big carton of smoothie. But I was shocked – there were two massive health-food stands full of all my favourite Lebanese food, like falafel and hummus. Who would have guessed a year ago that I would be eating hummus, something made from chickpeas? But I love it now – and chickpeas are really nutritious and full of protein. There was also raw veg juice readily available. Stuffed myself with loads of home-made salsa as a snack throughout the day.

I'd bought a couple of glasses of wine but couldn't touch them, because drinking in the day's a different thing from drinking at night. Everyone was downing beer and vodka, but having wine in the daytime is not something I can do any more.

Salsa with Veg

This is a great snack to dip into and so much better for you than the usual crisps and sweets!

250g (1 medium box) of cherry tomatoes, chopped
1 large garlic clove, peeled and crushed
half a red onion, finely chopped
2 tbsp fresh coriander, chopped
2 carrots, cut into thin strips
1 cucumber, cut into thin strips
2 sticks of celery, cut into thin strips

Place all the ingredients in a bowl and mix thoroughly.
    Cover and chill until ready to eat.

Sunday, 21 August 2005

Oh, holy shit. I'm never camping again. Call me a spoilt brat, call me a diva, call me whatever the hell you want, but if I ever buy a tent again it will have four bedrooms and an ensuite bathroom.

I was drinking water the entire time. The festival was amazing but I just can't deal with camping and can't wait to get home to my bed. The Portaloos were just . . . I couldn't even bring myself to use the showers. And this was in the VIP bit – which actually means nothing. It's just full of press.

It took us three hours to get home. Poor June was driving.

Tuesday, 23 August 2005

I got a text from Gillian yesterday saying I was ignoring her and that I needed to send her my food diaries every day. I've been doing this for eight months now. I don't keep a food diary every day.

Had to blitz my room completely today, as it was like a bomb site. Packed two suitcases, one for Ireland and one for Leeds, as I'm off to both places in the next few days.

This evening I went to meet all the guys from the *Pop Idol* production company Talkback for a quick drink. It was great, because most of them hadn't seen me in over a year and were amazed at the change in me. Then went to a Japanese restaurant with my friend Claire for dinner. Laura's moving out of the flat soon, so I also met up with her and her new flatmates, who were lovely. I was on the water.

Wednesday, 24 August 2005

Flew to Dublin to meet my friend Donna today, as we were going to the Franz Ferdinand / Scissor Sisters concert tonight.

God, how many people watched *You Are What You Eat?* Everyone at the concert was talking about it.

Thursday, 25 August 2005

Oh, what a beautiful morning,
Oh, what a beautiful day . . .

Donna's gone to work and left me in a five-star hotel.

I got up, went to the gym, had a shower and went down to this beach just outside Dublin for a few hours. There were wild horses running along the shore. It was unbelievable.

Had lunch and then paid 200 Euros for a two-hour massage. It was worth every penny. I was jelly when I got up.

A healthy dinner of halibut and steamed veg, and then home. This is the life.

Saturday, 27 August 2005

God, I'm dying. I was up at 6.30 a.m. to catch a flight to Leeds.

My friends Anne and Wayne – whose wedding I went to in April – were waiting for me. They took me home and I slept till 2 p.m. We had a barbecue tonight, but I wasn't drinking. I'm saving myself for tomorrow night.

Everyone was really jealous of the tuna I'd bought for the barbecue. And they ate all my salad. There was none left for me!

It's amazing. I've learned that people quite like healthy food. It's just that they think it takes ages to prepare. But cooking tuna on the barbecue takes the same amount of time as cooking a burger.

Monday, 29 August 2005

Last night I went to Escape, a complex of pubs in Leeds' town centre. Everyone was pissed when I got there – I had three glasses of wine in all and was absolutely plastered.

Hung-over today, but it's a Bank Holiday, so need to perk up.

Nic's mum, Jackie, is having a barbecue with lots of health food. Made my deliciously summery nut salad (see recipe on page 111) with barbecued salmon, which everyone loved. Am heading back to London later.

Tuesday, 30 August 2005

Aaargh. My first session with Dax for a month and I've really let myself go. After a music festival, a trip to Memphis and two trips to Dublin, everything is in agony. Dax has been away on holiday for a month too. I've been swimming and going to the gym, but nowhere near as intensively as I should have been. Measuring reveals I've lost four-and-a-half inches from my waist this month. I have, however, only lost 1 stone in three months.

This slowing-down business isn't good. I need to step it up and try to move up the levels on the cross-trainer.

Laura and I went to the restaurant down the road as it's her last night in the flat. I had a smoked-salmon salad. I'm very sad that Laura's leaving.

Thursday, 1 September 2005

I flew up to Manchester yesterday to the *Departure Lounge* studio to film the follow-up to Memphis. Brought a packed lunch with me, consisting of a salmon salad and a banana, two plums and a peach. Everyone was well impressed with my healthy food and I was quizzed as always about Gillian and her advice on dieting.

The filming went well and everyone was lovely up there. I did notice, though, that there were trays and trays of sandwiches left out that everyone was munching into all the time, just because they were there. If I hadn't been doing this healthy-eating plan I would have had a tray to myself. Note to self: don't go into TV.

Back working with Dax today and I'm in real agony, but it's great to be back in training.

I went to the theatre this evening and followed it with a Japanese meal – just love it. Had miso soup and chicken teriyaki with green beans. *You Are What You Eat* suggests staying clear of white rice or white noodles with these sorts of meals, but it's fine with brown rice or wholewheat noodles.

Saturday, 3 September 2005

I'm so tired. Ordered a lovely Rise and Shine juice – carrot, apple and ginger – from my hairdresser Richard Ward, and that woke me up.

I've been getting back into recording some tracks for a new album recently, which is really exciting – it's great being back in the studio again. I recorded a possible single, 'Breaking Free', in Townhouse Studios in west London today with Caroline and Jez, two professional songwriters, who've written some of the tracks. It went really well, but I'm still not sure if it's the single for me. I need to have some new material ready to present to record companies.

Rise and Shine Juice

Ginger provides an invigorating lift which, when combined with all the cleansing and digestive benefits of the carrot and the apple, gives a perfect kick-start to the morning.

4 carrots, washed, topped and tailed, and sliced
2 apples, washed, cored and sliced
1 small piece of ginger

Place all the ingredients in a juicer and juice thoroughly. Pour into a pint glass and serve with ice.

Monday, 5 September 2005

I went to meet Sam from *Pop Idol* for a drink and met his lovely girlfriend Ann. He said I looked amazing. Didn't drink at all.

Wednesday, 7 September 2005

Back to Dax Moy again today and Rick's just called to say that I need to go back to the studio to re-record two lines.

I did the vocal, but I probably should warm up more. The thing is that I think if you can sing, you can sing, and if you can't, you can't.

My career's completely in the lap of the gods now. I've done everything in my power to give this album the chance it needs. I've revamped my image. I've lost all the weight. If the album flops, I'll hold my head high and say to myself, 'Michelle, short of buying every copy of the album yourself, there's nothing else you could have done.'

No one will ever take away from me the fact that I won *Pop Idol*. No one will ever take away from me the fact that I was the first Scottish female ever to debut at Number One – I'm in the *Guinness World Records* for that. I've shown myself that I can lose all this weight and change my life. It doesn't matter what happens after that.

I've got a wad of cash in the bank, a house, a great life.

Now on my way to have my teeth cleaned. Then it's off to Margie for my colonic . . .

. . . after which, I feel a little queasy. The last twenty minutes were extremely painful: having your stomach filled with hot and cold water can give you cramps sometimes.

Sunday, 18 September 2005

I had friends arrive from Ireland last night and this morning I made a full Scottish breakfast for everyone, while I had a lovely fruit salad and a carrot, apple and ginger juice. They can't believe I can cook a fry-up without eating it. Am feeling very happy because last week Rick called to say that Sanctuary had given the thumbs up to managing me, which is fab.

Monday, 19 September 2005

I arrived in Glasgow for the premiere of *Goal!* and got my hair done. Then to Wagamama for food. Then back to the flat to get ready.

Everyone gasped when I came out of the room. I feel amazing. I'm wearing black to the premiere and no one's seen me in black for ages.

Oh, and the movie was ace.

Tuesday, 20 September 2005

Oh my God, I made it into the *Sun* newspaper. Full-length shot, and the headline was 'GOAL-DEN GIRL'. They said I was really sexy and looked great. I can't believe it. I've never been described as sexy by a paper. I cried, actually.

Went out with Carrie and another friend Mireille tonight. They both got shit-faced. I was surprisingly sober.

Wednesday, 21 September 2005

15 stone 11 pounds

Since the beginning of *You Are What You Eat*, I've lost 6 stone 1 pound.

The flight back to London is delayed. Never mind, I'm down to 15 stone 11 pounds and loving it.

Had some tuna stir-fry for dinner tonight – a good healthy midweek meal, nice and quick to prepare.

Tuna Stir-Fry

Made with fermented soy beans and darker in colour and flavour than soy sauce, tamari is a good alternative to teriyaki sauce, with a lower sodium content and no MSG. You can chop your own fresh vegetables if you have time, or 'cheat' and use one of those ready-prepared stir-fry bags if you're in a hurry. Stir-frying is a great way of cooking as it preserves many of the nutrients lost in boiling.

1 tuna steak
1 tsp of groundnut oil or other cooking oil
1 bag of fresh stir-fry vegetables (for example, chopped carrots, mushrooms, red peppers, beansprouts, baby corn, shredded cabbage, etc.)
3 tbsp of tamari sauce
2 tsp of Dijon mustard

Place the tuna steak under a preheated grill and cook for 5 minutes on each side. Meanwhile, lightly oil a wok and heat to a high temperature. Empty the bag of stir-fry vegetables into the wok, add the tamari sauce and cook quickly on a high heat for a couple of minutes, stirring constantly.

Once the tuna is cooked, spread the mustard on top of the steak and serve immediately with the stir-fried vegetables.

Saturday, 24 September 2005

After a couple of days of interviews and re-recording some vocals for a couple of new tracks on my album, I flew back to Spain yesterday for a short time away. Went to Donna's this evening for a barbecue as she has bought salmon and pumpkin seeds. How cool is that? Decided not to drink. My sister Maria did, however, and had to be put to bed.

Spain is not great news for sticking to the *You Are What You Eat* lifestyle plan. One day I walked for forty-five minutes trying to find health food. Like last time, it's out of season and the only restaurants open are dire Spanish places where the chicken's swimming in grease.

Since I'm generally drinking much less now, I'm also very self-conscious about being drunk at all as I'm sober around drunk people a lot more. I'm not perfect, though. Once, after having a few drinks with S in Spain, as far as I was concerned I was a stand-up comedienne / Ally McBeal rolled into one. For him I was probably a drunken psychopath whom he needed to get away from.

And I get drunk and lose control so quickly now. In the old days I could pack it away. I used to be never quite sober but never quite pissed either.

At least I don't seem to have put on any weight on holiday, though I haven't lost any either.

Thursday, 29 September 2005

I attended a breast cancer charity ball in Glasgow tonight. I had to ask for 'special dietary requirements' as they were serving creamy chicken in sauce. I might have loved that before – although I used to work in a hotel, so I know what they put in food for massive functions – but now I crave lemon, olive oil, garlicky tastes, that kind of thing. I was given melon to start with, followed by pumpkin soup, grilled sea bass and vegetables.

A great night and everyone thought I was looking fab.

Tuesday, 4 October 2005

I've been back in London for a couple of days, and going to the gym a lot.

In the evening I met up with Laura and Saira, a friend from Glasgow who's just moved to London. We went to the Spaghetti House and I had the most amazing salmon I've ever had in my life, with asparagus and cherry tomatoes.

Wednesday, 5 October 2005

Gym (again).

The girls – June, Saira and Laura – came round for dinner. I cooked a big pot of carrot and almond soup, and followed it with nut salad and peppers stuffed with goat's cheese, pine nuts and basil. It was a great laugh and June brought round this pink champagne that she'd bought in France, saying, 'Have a drink. Have a drink.'

So I had a tiny wee drop. It's the most heavenly drink I've ever tasted.

Thursday, 6 October 2005

I had an interview with BBC Radio Scotland, so was back up in Glasgow again today. Afterwards, I took my mum and the whole family out for dinner in Glasgow because I haven't spent proper quality time with them for a while.

We went to a lovely Italian restaurant. I had buffalo mozzarella to start with because it's not from cows, and I also ordered olives to share. My family always try bits of my dinner. Lynsey got so into my French onion soup that Tony, her boyfriend, said he was going to leave her if she made him another pot of it. Lynsey's also really into her soups now because of me.

They were all looking at my olives and I said, 'Try one.' Mum refused, but eventually tasted one and said it was disgusting. But she kept going back to them again.

French Onion Soup

Onions are believed to have all sorts of health benefits, including lowering cholesterol and blood pressure, and providing natural antibiotics and antioxidants.

1 tbsp of extra virgin olive oil
6 large red onions, peeled and chopped
2 tbsp of bouillon powder
1 garlic clove, crushed

Heat the oil gently in a large saucepan, then add the onions. Sauté on a very low heat for 5 to 10 minutes until the onions are soft. Half-fill the saucepan with water and add the remaining ingredients. Bring the soup to the boil and simmer for 10 to 15 minutes.

Friday, 7 October 2005

I'm still in Glasgow. Met Carrie in town at 2.30 p.m. We had
our hair done and got all glammed up for a fundraising gig in
Wick, an old Highland town right at the top of Scotland. Wick
was one of the first British cities to be bombed in daylight
during the Second World War, for no reason and without
warning. Fifteen people were killed and over half were children.
Unlike most places, though – places where there's a tourist
industry or more money – the bomb site hasn't been touched.
There's a hole in the ground full of fallen-down houses, bits of
old clothing and old-fashioned lampposts. It's a disgrace
because it should be a place of respect for the people who died,
but it's become a dumping ground. The BBC and a charity are
trying to raise money to turn the bomb site into a garden where
children can come and plant trees, and I was asked to come up
and do a benefit performance (Liz from Atomic Kitten is doing
one in Easterhouse in Glasgow next weekend). People are
paying a tenner a head – and they are squeezing 700 people in.

Anyway, we nearly didn't make it. We went to Central
Station to get the train to Inverness and Carrie said, 'Will we
have a wee glass of wine?'

I hadn't even had a sip before I realized we were in the
wrong train station. So Carrie and I were running through the
streets of Glasgow with our suitcases. We hadn't had a chance
to drink our wine and they weren't serving alcohol on the
train. I think it was a sign.

Had such a scream all the way up to Inverness, though.

Checked in to our hotel, which was beautiful, went down for
dinner and just as we passed reception, two full teams of shinty
(Scottish hurling) players checked in. Carrie and I almost fainted.

We said to one of the girls from the hotel, 'Are they all

going out tonight?' And she said, 'No, it's tomorrow night they all go out.' We were heartbroken.

Saturday, 8 October 2005

Arrived at Wick at 3.30 p.m. after a horrendous train journey. All they sold on the train was crisps, so we had to eat these nut bars of Carrie's. I missed my lunchbox.

It was a brill night, though. There was a question-and-answer session at the end, and someone asked how much weight I'd lost. I revealed it was six-and-a-half stone, and the whole place erupted.

I sang my three new tracks and 'From A Distance', and contributed my fee to the cause.

The fish up there was delicious and they put on fruit for me at breakfast because they knew I was a slave to Gillian McKeith. Back to London tomorrow.

Thursday, 13 October 2005

The Northern Line is not running so I had to get a taxi to Islington to see Dax, with the smelliest taxi driver in the entire world. It was death. I was hanging out the window and he asked me to close it because it was too cold. I just looked at him.

Went to Laura's for dinner and she made her fantastic miso soup. Then we sat there and man-bashed all evening with our friends Rachel and Jo. Apparently they too are working on a psycho table at the moment.

Then I came home to pack for Ireland.

Laura's Fantastic Miso Soup

(serves 4)

The 'instant' sachets of miso soup are great if you're in a hurry, but this recipe provides a heartier version using miso paste. It's still extremely quick and easy, though.

2 tbsp miso paste

1 medium onion, chopped

1 handful of mangetout, chopped

1 handful of bean sprouts

half a spring cabbage, shredded (or any other roughly
    chopped greens)

1 block of firm tofu

1 tsp vegetable bouillon powder (optional)

tamari sauce to taste (optional)

Bring a large saucepan of cold water to the boil. Once almost boiling, stir in the miso paste until it is fully dissolved, and add the chopped vegetables (you can use a bag of ready-to-cook stir-fry vegetables if you're in a hurry). Next, dry the tofu by patting it with kitchen roll and chop it into cubes. Add this to the soup as well, and simmer gently for 3 to 4 minutes. You might want to add a teaspoon of vegetable bouillon powder to taste. Serve in individual bowls, with some tamari sauce stirred in to taste if desired.

Monday, 17 October 2005

My friend Claire came round for dinner tonight, looking fantastic. We had a great laugh and she listened to the tracks on my new album and loved 'Everything Changes'.

I had to force a veggie juice down her throat but she actually loved it. It reminds me of myself during the first *You Are*

Fake 'Ferrero Rocher' Balls

Well, they might not fool the Ambassador, but these balls are a great healthy alternative to the usual chocolate treats. Dates are low in calories and high in iron and potassium. They're great if you suffer from anaemia, constipation or fatigue.

1 handful of mixed nuts (unsalted)
24 dates, stoned
2 tsp of crushed almonds
juice of 1 lime

Place the nuts into a blender or food processor and blend thoroughly until they form small crumbs. Pour onto a large plate and leave to one side. Next blend the dates, almonds and lime juice together until the mixture resembles a mound of dough. Remove from the blender, and, using your hands, separate the dough into approximately 6 to 8 pieces. Shape into balls then roll in the crushed nuts to coat. Put the finished balls onto a clean plate and chill for an hour in the fridge before serving.

What You Eat programme, when I said avocado was the devil's fruit and Gillian made me an avocado juice heavily disguised with lime. I surprised myself by liking it too. I made Claire baked salmon and then some of my fake 'Ferrero Rocher' balls.

Tuesday, 18 October 2005

I met Kim from *Pop Idol* at Clapham Junction for lunch. Gave her some of my designer clothes because they're all too big for me. She's lost a lot of weight too – mainly by exercising – and she's just one size above me now. A nice girly day.

Wednesday, 19 October 2005

I'm loving the November issue of *You Are What You Eat* magazine's 'Flame-grilled Whoppers' – Alex Gazzola's piece that exposes dietary myths. My favourite myths are:

- 'Diet drinks are good for you' – FALSE. 'Diet drinks make you fat, in my view,' says Mike Irvine, nutritionist and personal trainer. Apparently, they create carbohydrate cravings that people eventually give in to.
- 'Olive oil has fewer calories than butter' – FALSE. Olive oil is still 100 per cent fat and has just as many calories as other fats, and more than butter, which is 80 per cent fat.
- 'Celery has negative calories' – FALSE. Although it has very few calories, it's not true that it takes more calories to chew and digest than it actually contains.
- 'Grapefruit dissolves body fat' – FALSE. Did anyone really believe this?

- 'Only water counts towards your daily intake of fluid' – FALSE. All fluids count towards your daily intake of water, even tea and coffee (though you're advised to drink these in moderation).
- 'Eating food late at night is more fattening than if you eat it earlier in the evening' – FALSE. Your body is burning calories all the time – even when you're sleeping.
- 'White spots on your nails always means you have calcium deficiency' – FALSE. Sometimes they are just caused by a common trauma to the nail.

Thursday, 20 October 2005

Whoops. I missed the gasman this morning – just slept through him. The landlord will kill me. He left a message weeks ago on my landline to tell me he was coming, but who uses their landline? I don't even know what my number is.

On the plus side, I've lost 4 pounds this week.

To the hairdresser's this afternoon, as I went to Anna Scholz's launch party for her new collection at the Sanderson Hotel this evening.

I had a fab time and everyone was so complimentary about my new figure. They were having a laugh with me and saying I wasn't a role model for big women any more. I had about six glasses of pink champagne with Laura. (Who can refuse pink champagne?) And I didn't eat the pink chocolate love hearts, for God's sake.

We tried to be really good and leave at 10 o'clock, but we went past the bar downstairs and there was just a sea of the most gorgeous, rich men, all in Savile Row suits. So Laura and I were like, 'We're not going anywhere.'

We got straight in there and ordered two Cosmopolitans and a bottle of water, and it came to £36! I thought, 'These men in here have got to be padded.' We got a lot of attention because we were the only two girls in there and we were all dolled up for the launch party.

We ended up rolling home steaming at 12.30. Oops.

Monday, 24 October 2005

Well, this weekend turned into a bit of a big one. After Anna Scholz's launch party on Thursday, I suffered all day on Friday with a hangover, not helped by having a driving lesson and a Brazilian wax. Never get waxed when you're hung-over because you feel everything. Usually I can cope with the pain, but this time I had tears streaming down my face. Anyway, that night we went to Abacus, my favourite bar in the City. I'm afraid that turned into a bit of a bender too. And then yesterday, my friend Neil had organized a corporate day at Upton Park, West Ham's ground. There was a big box with free food and booze.

I went along saying, 'I'm not going to drink. I'm not going to drink. I'm not going to drink.' And I had my first glass of wine at midday and didn't eat all day, which is horrendous. I kept thinking, 'I'll get something later' and never did. And again, I was steaming by the end of the evening.

Somehow, despite all this heavy drinking, I've managed to lose 2 pounds since I last weighed myself. That's me done with booze, though, at least for another six months. As much as I love seeing my friends and occasionally getting drunk, three days in quick succession is too much. That's not something I'm proud of. Even as I was doing it I knew what was coming. It was just that there were these three important occasions . . . but that's a crap excuse. I don't think I can do it again, though. I'm getting too old for it.

Spent all day doing a lot of walking, and drinking and eating raw vegetable juices and fruit to make up for it. I don't crave classic hangover cures like fry-ups any more. Just good stuff. I couldn't sleep last night for thinking about carrot juice.

Got a hangover? Have two bananas. You'll feel amazing.

Wednesday, 26 October 2005

Laura's birthday, she's thirty-one.

I arrived at a photo shoot for *Woman's Own* slightly late this afternoon as I had to pick up Kaiser Chiefs tickets from the post office. The magazine asked me to bring my own clothes and I was happy with that – I've bought loads of new ones recently because I've lost so much weight and none of my old clothes fit me. It was quick and painless. They're printing a piece about me and my weight loss in January.

We were out for Laura's birthday tonight but I wasn't drinking – it's my second driving test tomorrow.

Friday, 28 October 2005

I failed my test again yesterday. Oh no! But the examiner said I was unlucky and should apply again straight away.

It was the Kaiser Chiefs concert last night. I only had a few glasses of wine but feel rough today – I suppose they *were* pint glasses . . .

Had a major meeting with a record company today. The guy said, 'I really like your look. Quite grungy.' I felt like telling him I hadn't been to bed and had been at a rock concert, but I didn't.

To Glasgow now, so I'm shooting off to Euston station. I'm really looking forward to the break.

Sunday, 30 October 2005

To Tesco, where I spent £161 on food, because all my family are coming for dinner. That's the thing about healthy eating. It is more expensive, at least the way I do it, but maybe that says more about my spending habits. And I always buy organic. People say different things about organic food. If you buy organic you won't consume the remains of any pesticides or fertilizers, but some say that our body is perfectly able to deal with and detoxify these things in small amounts. Others say it's worth buying organic because it's simply more nutritious – wild or organic fish is definitely more healthy than farmed. I think I'll carry on in that case. But even if organic isn't easily available, the most important thing is to eat fruit and veg, full stop – even non-organic stuff. I put on the most gorgeous buffet: smoked salmon on a bed of lettuce, stir-fried tofu with green beans, that kind of thing. And they all *loved* it.

I played them my new songs, but don't know if they liked them that much. They all just sort of sat there. My family want to hear me singing big power ballads, and these new ones are really rocky.

Monday, 31 October 2005

Flew back to London, for a very busy day.

I met Sarah the stylist, who Celador have brought in for the show; she was really lovely. It's a nervous thing meeting a new stylist. My usual stylist is Faye, but she's got no time just now because she's working so hard on *The X Factor*.

I was very nervous because I know I've lost a lot of weight, but I'm still not sure that I've got the figure for designer clothes. But Celador are adamant I'm going to do a red-carpet event in a designer dress and want me to attend the Variety Club Awards on 13 November. It's going to be the climax of the *You Are What You Eat* show. The fact is that I am a size 16 now, but a size 16 for these couture labels is different to what it means to everyone else. You still have to be toned and have a particular figure to get away with it. I don't have that yet. I've still got this loose skin where I've lost the weight but my skin hasn't yet tightened up.

I left feeling quite deflated.

Tuesday, 1 November 2005

Up at 8.30 a.m., as I'm filming all day with *You Are What You Eat*. Today we went to designer Frank Usher and found the most gorgeous turquoise dress for the awards ceremony. It needs to be taken in slightly and a little jacket has to be made to cover up the tops of my arms, as I still don't feel comfortable showing them. The dress is covered in tiny, delicate little pleats, which I thought would look awful on me when I put it on, but they didn't move. It's really flattering.

So Celador were right. I *can* get away with wearing a designer dress after all. I'm ecstatic. This is definitely the beginning of a new era for me.

Went to Townhouse Studios to do some more recording in the afternoon.

All in all a fab day, topped off with a Japanese meal.

Wednesday, 2 November 2005

Today I gutted the house from top to bottom, and worked up more of a sweat than I ever have in the gym.

Then a big shop at Sainsbury's as Laura, Saira and June are coming over for dinner. Made a lovely vegetable soup, followed by chestnut roast – one of Gillian's recipes. It went down a treat. The girls were so impressed. It was one of those cold autumn nights and I fed them good, hearty, warming food. Got a round of applause.

Thursday, 3 November 2005

Gillian just called to tell me that there's a rumour going around all the magazines that I've started to put a lot of weight back on, and that I'm off the *You Are What You Eat* healthy-eating regime and off the wagon. I rang her back asking her to be more specific about who said this, because as far as I know the magazines have all been great to me.

I've told her if she doesn't reveal her sources I'll think she's making it up!

Saturday, 5 November 2005

Went out with a load of *Pop Idol* researchers on Thursday whom I hadn't seen for ages. They ordered two huge plates of nachos and just couldn't believe it when I refused them. Nachos used to be my favourite food and the ones I made were world-renowned. They would be loaded down with a full block of cheese, sour cream and salsa. Now, just thinking about them makes me feel bloated.

People who haven't done something life-changing like the *You Are What You Eat* plan can't see why I don't allow myself the odd nacho, but because my body has been reprogrammed I don't even feel the urge to eat stuff like that – and I'm not turning back now. Not after having come this far. And when friends tell you how good you've been it spurs you on. Like everyone, I love being commended. It also reminds you of how you've taken control. I didn't touch a drop of drink that night either because I didn't want to.

Yesterday was spent at the London Weekend Television studios with Sarah, my stylist for the Variety Club Awards on the 13th – next Sunday. The beautiful blue designer dress I'm going to be wearing needed taking in around the bust, and the straps have been shortened. Taking the bust in worked in my favour. My boobs look humungous now!

The whole outfit is like something from a fairy tale. As I was trying it on, a load of models from *This Morning*, which was being broadcast live in the same building, kept running in and out saying, 'Oh my God, you look so gorgeous!' And I was saying, 'No, *you* look gorgeous!'

Went to a bonfire party in north London tonight. June and I took an hour and a half to get to it because we didn't know where we were going. They don't have any signposts in north

London to keep the south Londoners out. We'd already eaten Lebanese before we got there (vine leaves, falafel, hummus) because we'd been forewarned that there would be traditional Bonfire Night food there – sausages, jacket potatoes with cheese, that sort of thing. Believe it or not, it's fine eating beforehand and making your own preparations. It's just a habit that you get into like any other. We didn't drink either. We didn't need to. Like kids, we were already overexcited because there were going to be fireworks.

Tuesday, 8 November 2005

Filmed for December's *You Are What You Eat* with Dax yesterday. The crew were all well impressed at how fit I am. I was working really hard doing kickboxing and I was hardly sweating at all.

Dax was really generous. He kept saying how far I'd come and how much fitter I was than a lot of his clients who were much thinner than me. He also made an interesting point about the BMI – Body Mass Index – and how it's not always a reliable indicator of health, fitness or obesity. The BMI uses a calculation involving a person's weight and height together, and height is included because the thinking is that a healthy weight for one person is different for someone else who is taller or shorter. Dax is a very fit man and doesn't have an ounce of body fat on him, yet according to the BMI scale his weight – 15 stone – in conjunction with his height makes him obese. Something's obviously wrong there.

Had the photo shoot for the book cover today and I'm very excited because it's at Holborn Studios, which is where a lot of stuff for *Pop Idol* was shot. The smell of it sends me right back to that amazing time. It felt really strange to be there on my own though, without the other eleven *Pop Idol* contestants running through the corridors. But this time it was a different group of people there. I guess things move on.

Lindsey, who works for Faye, my stylist, brought the most amazing clothes in for the shoot. I was five dress sizes bigger when she last dressed me. Lindsey was shocked. Some of the size 16 tops were even too big and I had to wear size 14.

The pictures turned out brilliantly. I think the difference between me now and me then, before the *You Are What You Eat* plan and before I decided to live a healthier lifestyle, is unbelievable. It never ceases to amaze me. The photographer was amazing and took fab pictures. He was like Austin Powers – 'Oh yeah, baby.' I thought, 'This is a diet book, not *FHM*. Calm down!' But he was great.

Saturday, 12 November 2005

On Thursday I had my final styling meeting with Sarah for the Variety Club Awards. She's found me these beautiful diamanté Gina shoes (with five-and-a-half-inch heels) and a matching bag. I feel like a proper princess. All the final adjustments have been made and the dress and the cape are just gorgeous.

Another quiet night in tonight. I'm really not in the mood for going out or drinking just now because of that wild long weekend I had three weeks ago. I think I sickened myself with drink. I felt so poisoned, and that feeling's lasted. My mates were calling me tonight saying, 'Come out, come out, come out,' and I could think of nothing worse. It's a physical and a mental thing. I felt so guilty with myself after that weekend because it was the first time I'd done it since starting the regime. I think I'll have to tell Gillian I've been drinking again the next time we're filming. I'm sure I won't come out alive, but this book can be my memorial.

Again, I like the control of not drinking. I like saying to myself, 'OK, you've had a wild weekend, but you're not slipping back into your old ways again. You're not doing that again until Christmas.' If I can – and want to – stand it at Christmas, that is. If I don't want to drink, I won't drink. More than anything, I want to hang on to this energy that I've had ever since I first detoxed – and alcohol saps that. I'm also loving the fact that I've not had a beginning-of-winter flu this year, which I've always had before. And I can't remember the last time I had a cold – I used to get them all the time.

Yesterday I began the final preparations to be ready for the Variety Club Awards. I visited Dax at the gym and then Sean at Richard Ward's salon to have my hair coloured. As if that wasn't exciting enough, Sean's going to get me and Lynsey tickets for the launch party of the Take That Greatest Hits CD. Lynsey was Take That's biggest fan ever – she had to call the helpline when they broke up. As soon as I told her about the launch party she asked Dad to get her old posters down from the loft and started listening to all their albums again.

Tonight Laura and I stayed in and chilled, covered in St. Tropez. Now I'm starting to get nervous about tomorrow night. It's the first red-carpet event I've done since I lost all the weight. I've been to the gym more times this week than usual, and for longer, and done some extra sit-ups just to be sure that I look shit-hot. Laura drank a whole bottle of wine on her own and was hilarious. I asked her how different she felt aged thirty-one from when she was twenty-five. She said she spent her entire twenties being paranoid about Visible Panty Lines and now she's like, 'I've got a knicker line. Deal with it.'

Off to bed now for some beauty sleep. Brian Ormond arrives from Ireland in the morning to escort me to the awards.

Sunday, 13 November 2005: Variety Club Awards Day

The *You Are What You Eat* crew arrived at the flat at 2 p.m. to interview me and to set up a camera to film the preparations for the big night. The interview forces me to think about the journey and how far I've come this year and, to be totally honest, I'm feeling as pleased as punch with myself. The camera crew leave to find a proper cup of tea because all I give them is herbal tea and they're sick of it. Sarah the stylist and Lee the make-up artist arrive to complete my transformation.

By four o'clock I'm feeling really nervous because things aren't moving very quickly and I'm thinking, 'It's nearly time. It's nearly time. I just want to look perfect.' Lee is fabulous. I'm not sure whether you're supposed to admit to these things or not, but after spending three hours in make-up I just feel beautiful – apart from my hair, which looks like I've been dragged through a hedge backwards. And, all this time I'm thinking, 'The *You Are What You Eat* journey ends here. I'm on my own now. Will I be able to do this on my own?' But it's only the filming that stops here, and my relationship with the show. What mustn't stop – and won't stop – is the way I live my life these days: healthy and happy and in control. That's not going to change.

Lee straightens my hair and sends me to look in the mirror. I can't believe it. I look so different. I've lost so much weight and I look so much healthier. If ever I needed a visual of what I've achieved, it's there, looking back at me from the mirror. I'm still scared, but I really want to do the red carpet now, the show, all of it.

The car arrives – a black Merc – and we're away. James the director has warned me that there will be a lot of paparazzi at the event, and said Celador would be filming me walking up the red carpet. Brian is holding my hand in the car and he can feel it shaking.

'You're so nervous. What's wrong with you?' he says.

'I've not been on a red carpet for a year and a half. Are they going to notice any difference? Why am I putting myself out there? Maybe I shouldn't bother.'

I tell him that Louis Walsh said in the paper a couple of months ago that he wasn't particularly a fan of mine, but that I was his favourite Scottish group (geddit?). But he didn't stop there. He went on to say that I was the only woman he knew who could lose several stone and still look hugely fat.

Brian tells me that I shouldn't take any notice of him. Then he reminds me of the recent *heat* piece which was very supportive and full of admiration that I'd lost 8 entire stone – a massive amount. It even carried pictures with a big caption saying, 'Look!' More people read *heat* than listen to Louis Walsh, I'm sure of that.

When we arrive, I can hear the paparazzi calling my name from down the road – 'Michelle, Michelle.' Then the car stops and I step out on to the pavement and all hell breaks loose. 'Michelle, Michelle, Michelle!' 'Look to the right!' 'Look to the left!' 'Over here!' Flashlights are going off everywhere and I think to myself, 'Well done, girl.'

I remember what I've been taught by all the stylists that I've worked with, and I look at the photographers straight on and then twist my shoulders and body to the left slightly, keeping my shoulders back. All the time I'm thinking, '*Pleeeease* let these pictures look good in the morning. Please let them do me justice.' But I've done it. I'm standing on a red carpet in a designer dress having lost all the weight I wanted to and feeling a million dollars inside and out. 'I've lost 8 stone,' I think again, and it is still an incredible thought.

I'm sitting on a table with Carol Vorderman who looks fantastic, and she's with Richard Whiteley's partner, Kathryn. Also sitting here is Catherine bleeding Tate! I can't believe it's her. And she's just come running up to me saying, 'Oh my God! I loved you on *Pop Idol*. I voted for you.'

Am I bovvered? Yes I am. I can't believe I'm here.

Then, the biggest deal of all. Brian has seen Simon Cowell – whom he knows from being on *Pop Idol*, of course – and he's about to go and say hi to him. Simon's sitting on Max Clifford's table, and my first instinct is to stay away. Simon was rude about me in the press, but then again he's the pantomime baddie and he knows I know it.

But Brian is already off and Simon seems genuinely delighted to see him. He must have asked Brian who he's with because at that moment they both turn to face me and Simon's face brightens up even more and he calls me over. I'm disappointed that he still has this power over me, but I feel myself drawn towards his table. I have a weird feeling of a circle closing; at the beginning there was *Pop Idol* and Simon Cowell, and two years on, with my life and health so different – so much better – here he is again.

'Oh my God, Michelle! Hey gorgeous.' Big kiss. 'You look stunning. You've lost so much weight. You look beautiful.'

It's true. The journey was worth every step. And it's only just beginning.

Appendix
INTEGRATED MOVEMENT TRAINING

Integrated Movement Training, created by Dax Moy, is a system of training that takes into account the functional roles of the various muscles and joints of the body.

This short routine only lasts about ten minutes, but by the end you'll have exercised all 600 muscles of the body across every joint and in all possible directions. Repeated use of these exercises, along with regular and consistent exercise in your daily life, will result in you becoming stronger, more toned and more supple.

The aim of Integrated Movement Training is to provide a full and thorough preparation for activity. The exercises chosen provide optimal neural, muscular and skeletal stimulation, allowing for an increase in stability, strength, power and flexibility while reducing the risk of injury associated with many forms of conditioning.

Note: it is important that posture remains in alignment throughout all Integrated Movement Training exercises. *Please consult your doctor if you are attempting exercise for the first time, particularly if you are seriously overweight, pregnant, elderly or infirm, or suffering from any injuries or illnesses.*

For Exercises 1 to 9, the start position is to stand tall with a good posture and belly button slightly pulled in. Feet should be hip-width apart and the knees soft (i.e. not locked). Shoulders should be back and down.

Exercises 1 to 5 should be performed using a small handweight or medicine ball.

Exercise 1

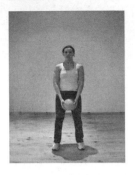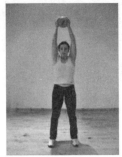

Adopt the start position, holding the weight with both hands. Keeping arms straight and maintaining a straight posture, raise the weight directly overhead and back to the start position for 5 repetitions.

Exercise 2

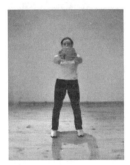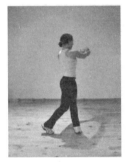

Adopt the start position. Hold the weight straight out in front of you at shoulder level using both hands. Keeping your arms straight and maintaining a straight spine, bring the weight across your body and gradually add a rotation from the hips, and return to the start position, for 5 repetitions. Repeat on the other side of the body.

Exercise 3

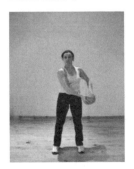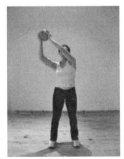

Adopt the start position, holding the weight with both hands. Keeping your arms straight and maintaining a straight spine, raise your arms diagonally overhead from the left hip and back to the start position for 5 repetitions. Repeat on the other side of the body.

Exercise 4

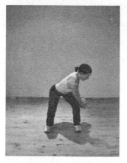
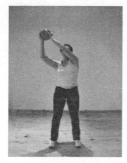

Adopt the start position, holding the weight with both hands. Keeping your arms straight and maintaining a straight spine, bend slightly to lower the weight to the outside of your left knee. Now, raise your arms diagonally overhead from the left knee and back to the start position for 5 repetitions. Repeat on the other side of the body.

Exercise 5

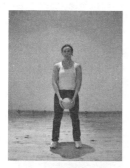
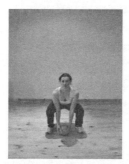
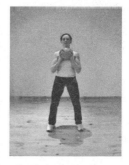

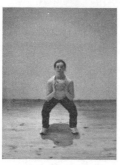
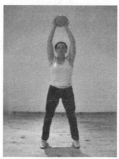

1. Adopt the start position, holding the weight with both hands. Push your bottom back and perform a squat, reaching down to the floor with the weight. Make sure your bodyweight is back and your knees do not move in front of your toes.

2. Maintaining a straight spine, stand up while bringing the weight to your chest, then perform a second squat with the weight in this new position.

3. As you rise from the squat, press the weight overhead in a fluid motion before returning to the start position. Repeat the sequence for 10 repetitions.

Exercise 6

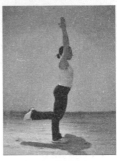 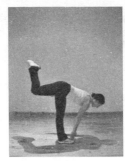

1. Adopt the start position. Stand on your left leg with your right arm fully extended above your head.
2. Maintaining the straight spine as best you can, reach forward with your right hand to touch your left foot, while keeping your left leg straight.
3. Perform 10 repetitions and then repeat on the other side, using the opposing leg and arm.

Exercise 7

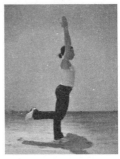 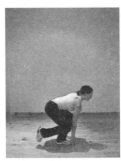

1. Adopt the start position. Stand on your left leg with your right arm fully extended above your head.
2. Maintaining the straight spine as best you can, reach forward with your right hand to touch your left foot, this time bending your left knee.
3. Perform 10 repetitions and then repeat on the other side, using the opposing leg and arm.

Exercise 8

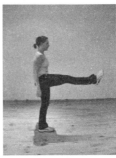 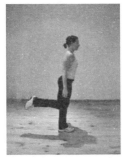

1. Adopt the start position. Put your weight on your left leg and swing your right leg forward under control to a comfortable height.
2. As your right leg returns and passes the supporting leg, bend your right knee as depicted.
3. Gradually increase the height, speed and force of the movement for 10 repetitions, and then repeat on the other leg.

Exercise 9

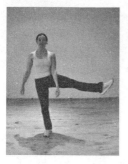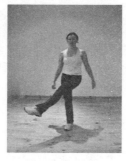

1. Adopt the start position. Put your weight on your left leg and swing your right leg from left to right in front of your body. Point your toes in the direction that your leg is travelling.
2. Gradually increase the height, speed and force of the movement for 10 repetitions, and then repeat for the other leg.

Exercise 10

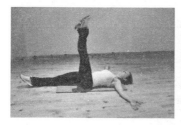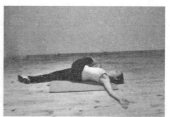

1. Lie flat on your back with your arms at 90 degrees to your body, and your legs straight out in front of you. Raise your left leg vertically.
2. Slowly lower the leg down and across toward your right hand, hold for 2 seconds and then return to the start position, for 10 repetitions. Repeat for the other leg.

Exercise 11

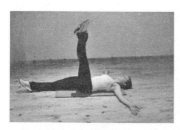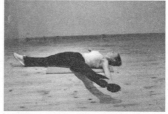

1. Lie flat on your back with your arms at 90 degrees to your body, and your legs straight out in front of you. Raise your left leg vertically.
2. Slowly lower the leg down and across toward your *left* hand, hold for 2 seconds and then return to the start position, for 10 repetitions. Repeat for the other leg.

Exercise 12

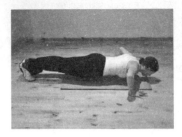 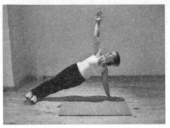

1. Adopt a push-up position keeping your back flat, feet together and tummy muscles slightly pulled in.
2. Slowly lower your chest to the floor and then press up to arms' length.
3. At the top, rotate your body and reach your right hand up. Look up at the palm of your hand, and hold for 2 seconds, and then return to the push-up position. Repeat 5 times, then do the same on the other side.

INDEX

carbohydrate–protein
combinations in 75, 124, 172
carbonated drinks 94
celery 201
cheese 52, 103
dates 200
diet drinks 201
eggs 74, 83
80:20 rule of 113
essential fatty acids in 145
fish 68, 74, 80, 90, 131–2, 149,
175, 193
fruit 75, 78
fruit and vegetable juices 95–7
ginger 109, 190
grapefruit 201
hemp seed 110
honey 74
Lebanese 124
Japanese 144–5
mangoes 127, 170
meat 74, 75, 90
milk 74, 90
miso 124–5, 199
nachos 208
nuts 74, 83, 90, 111, 125, 200
olive oil 201
onions 196
oranges 127
organic 205
potatoes 73
processed 52, 75
quinoa 124
refined carbohydrates 72–3
rules concerning 72–9
salt 71, 74
seaweed 126
seeds 125
sex life linked to 170
sushi 145
tamari 193
turkey 143
vegetables 75
water 79, 202
wholegrain and wholemeal
products 72–3
yoghurt 74
see also detox: foods allowed and
forbidden during; detox: typical
menu for; recipes; *You Are What
You Eat*
Fox, Dr 10
Fuller, Simon 39–40, 57, 59

Garrett, Lesley 32
Gates, Gareth 21
Gee, Kim 24, 25, 47, 201
Gervais, Ricky 176
G4 146
GMTV 162
Goody, Jade 29
grapefruit juice 96
Green Day 117

Harrison, Ann 147, 148
heat 143, 153–4, 213
Hendry, Sharon 31
herbal teas, *see* teas
Hide, Chris 25, 102
Houston, Whitney 151

InStyle 171, 176, 177
Integrated Movement Training
215–20
Ita (director) 67, 123

Jackie (friend's mother) 140, 188
James (director) 213
Jo (friend) 198
John (voice coach) 26
Jordan 29
June (friend) 71, 103, 105, 124, 130,
144, 170–1, 195, 207, 208

Kelly, Lorraine 162–3

Laura (friend) 44, 61, 71, 88, 89, 95,
110, 119–20, 138, 155, 186,
189, 195, 198, 207, 211
thirty-first birthday of 204
Lee (make-up artist) 212
Linda (colonic-irrigation
practitioner) 135
Linda (friend) 44, 71, 122, 123
Lindsey (stylist) 210
Lisa (make-up artist) 127
London bombings 171
Ludwig (friend) 146, 165

MacAulay, Fred 160
McKeith, Gillian 16, 57, 61, 62–5,
71, 72, 81–4, 95, 104, 112–13,
128, 131, 161–2, 207
initial doubts of 168
meditation recommended by 172
Michelle's celebratory dinner
with 167